Stress and Immune-Based Diseases

Guest Editor

GAILEN D. MARSHALL Jr, MD, PhD

IMMUNOLOGY AND ALLERGY CLINICS OF NORTH AMERICA

www.immunology.theclinics.com

Consulting Editor
RAFEUL ALAM, MD, PhD

February 2011 • Volume 31 • Number 1

SAUNDERS an imprint of ELSEVIER, Inc.

W.B. SAUNDERS COMPANY

A Division of Elsevier Inc.

1600 John F. Kennedy Blvd., • Suite 1800 • Philadelphia, PA 19103-2899.

http://www.theclinics.com

IMMUNOLOGY AND ALLERGY CLINICS OF NORTH AMERICA Volume 31, Number 1
February 2011 ISSN 0889–8561, ISBN-13: 978-1-4557-0460-6

Editor: Patrick Manley

Immunology and Allergy Clinics of North America (ISSN 0889–8561) is published quarterly by Elsevier Inc., 360 Park Avenue South, New York, NY 10010-1710. Months of issue are February, May, August, and November. Periodicals postage paid at New York, NY and additional mailing offices. Subscription prices are $272.00 per year for US individuals, $392.00 per year for US institutions, $129.00 per year for US students and residents, $334.00 per year for Canadian individuals, $187.00 per year for Canadian students, $486.00 per year for Canadian institutions, $379.00 per year for international individuals, $486.00 per year for international institutions, $187.00 per year for international students. To receive student/resident rate, orders must be accompanied by name of affiliated institution, date of term, and the *signature* of program/residency coordinator on institution letterhead. Orders will be billed at individual rate until proof of status is received. Foreign air speed delivery is included in all *Clinics* subscription prices. All prices are subject to change without notice. **POSTMASTER:** Send address changes to *Immunology and Allergy Clinics of North America,* Elsevier Health Sciences Division, Subscription Customer Service, 3251 Riverport Lane, Maryland Heights, MO 63043. **Customer Service: 1-800-654-2452 (U.S. and Canada); 314-447-8871 (outside U.S. and Canada). Fax: 314-447-8029. E-mail: journalscustomerservice-usa@elsevier.com (for print support); journalsonlinesupport-usa@elsevier.com (for online support).**

Reprints. For copies of 100 or more, of articles in this publication, please contact the Commercial Reprints Department, Elsevier Inc., 360 Park Avenue South, New York, New York 10010-1710. Tel. (212) 633-3812, Fax: (212) 462-1935, e-mail: reprints@elsevier.com.

Immunology and Allergy Clinics of North America is covered in MEDLINE/PubMed (Index Medicus), Current Contents/Life Sciences, Science Citation Index, ISI/BIOMED, Chemical Abstracts, and EMBASE/Excerpta Medica.

Printed and bound by CPI Group (UK) Ltd, Croydon, CR0 4YY

Transferred to Digital Print 2011

Contributors

CONSULTING EDITOR

RAFEUL ALAM, MD, PhD
Veda and Chauncey Ritter Chair in Immunology, Professor and Director, Division
of Immunology and Allergy, National Jewish Health; and University of Colorado
Health Sciences Center, Denver, Colorado

GUEST EDITOR

GAILEN D. MARSHALL Jr, MD, PhD
Professor of Medicine and Pediatrics; Vice Chair for Research; Chief, Laboratory
of Behavioral Immunology Research; Director, Division of Clinical Immunology
and Allergy, Department of Medicine, University of Mississippi Medical Center,
Jackson, Mississippi

AUTHORS

SANDEEP K. AGARWAL, MD, PhD
Assistant Professor of Medicine, Division of Rheumatology and Clinical Immunogenetics,
Department of Internal Medicine, University of Texas Health Science Center at Houston
(UTHSC-H), Houston, Texas

REBECCA G. ALLEN, BS
Division of Oral Biology, College of Dentistry; Institute for Behavioral Medicine Research;
Graduate Student, Integrated Biomedical Sciences Graduate Program,
The Ohio State University College of Medicine, Columbus, Ohio

MICHAEL T. BAILEY, PhD
Assistant Professor, Division of Oral Biology, College of Dentistry; Institute for Behavioral
Medicine Research, The Ohio State University College of Medicine, Columbus, Ohio

EDITH CHEN, PhD
Associate Professor of Psychology, Department of Psychology, University of British
Columbia, Vancouver, British Columbia, Canada

ERIN S. COSTANZO, PhD
Assistant Professor, Department of Psychiatry, Carbone Comprehensive Cancer Center,
University of Wisconsin-Madison, Madison, Wisconsin

NINABAHEN D. DAVE, MBBS
Clinical Fellow, Laboratory of Behavioral Immunology Research, Division of Clinical
Immunology and Allergy, Department of Medicine, University of Mississippi Medical
Center, Jackson, Mississippi

JEAN-PHILIPPE GOUIN, MA
Clinical Psychology PhD Candidate, Department of Psychology, The Ohio State
University; Institute for Behavioral Medicine Research, The Ohio State University College
of Medicine, Columbus, Ohio

KATHI L. HEFFNER, PhD
Assistant Professor of Psychiatry, Department of Psychiatry, The Rochester Center
for Mind-Body Research, University of Rochester Medical Center, Rochester, New York

AMY R. HUFNAGLE, BS
Graduate Student, Division of Oral Biology, College of Dentistry; Institute for Behavioral
Medicine Research, The Ohio State University College of Medicine, Columbus, Ohio

JANICE K. KIECOLT-GLASER, PhD
Distinguished University Professor; S. Robert Davis Chair of Medicine; Professor
of Psychiatry and Psychology, Department of Psychology, The Ohio State University;
Institute for Behavioral Medicine Research; Department of Psychiatry, The Ohio State
University College of Medicine, Columbus, Ohio

SUSAN K. LUTGENDORF, PhD
Professor, Departments of Psychology, Urology, Obstetrics and Gynecology,
Holden Comprehensive Cancer Center, University of Iowa, Iowa City, Iowa

GAILEN D. MARSHALL Jr, MD, PhD
Professor of Medicine and Pediatrics; Vice Chair for Research; Chief, Laboratory
of Behavioral Immunology Research; Director, Division of Clinical Immunology
and Allergy, Department of Medicine, University of Mississippi Medical Center,
Jackson, Mississippi

COURTNEY J. MCCRAY, MD
Division of Rheumatology and Clinical Immunogenetics, Department of Internal Medicine,
University of Texas Health Science Center at Houston (UTHSC-H), Houston, Texas

GREGORY E. MILLER, PhD
Associate Professor of Psychology, Department of Psychology, University of British
Columbia, Vancouver, British Columbia, Canada

NICOLE D. POWELL, PhD
Research Scientist, Division of Oral Biology, College of Dentistry; Institute for Behavioral
Medicine Research, The Ohio State University College of Medicine, Columbus, Ohio

KRISTINA E. REHM, PhD
Postdoctoral Research Fellow, Laboratory of Behavioral Immunology Research, Division
of Clinical Immunology and Allergy, Department of Medicine, University of Mississippi
Medical Center, Jackson, Mississippi

HANNAH M.C. SCHREIER, MA
PhD Student, Department of Psychology, University of British Columbia, Vancouver,
British Columbia, Canada

JOHN F. SHERIDAN, PhD
Associate Dean for Research, and George C. Paffenbarger Professor, Division of Oral
Biology, College of Dentistry; Institute for Behavioral Medicine Research; Integrated
Biomedical Sciences Graduate Training Program, The Ohio State University
College of Medicine, Columbus, Ohio

ANIL K. SOOD, MD
Professor, Departments of Gynecologic Oncology, Cancer Biology, and Center for RNA Interference and Non-Coding RNA, MD Anderson Cancer Center, University of Texas, Houston, Texas

ROSALIND J. WRIGHT, MD, MPH
Associate Professor of Medicine, Channing Laboratory, Department of Medicine, Brigham and Women's Hospital, Harvard Medical School; Department of Environmental Health, Harvard School of Public Health, Boston, Massachusetts

LIANBIN XIANG, MD
Assistant Professor of Medicine, Laboratory of Behavioral Immunology Research, Division of Clinical Immunology and Allergy, Department of Medicine, University of Mississippi Medical Center, Jackson, Mississippi

Contents

assessing the effects of psychological stress on asthma outcomes and discusses the benefits and disadvantages of different measures for assessing stress, including subjective questionnaires, event checklists, and interview-based approaches. We discuss the importance of taking into account the timing and chronicity of stress, as well as individuals' subjective appraisals of stress. We suggest that, although questionnaire and checklist approaches are easier to administer, interview-based stress assessments are preferable, where feasible, because they generate richer and more in-depth information regarding the stressors that people experience. In addition, this kind of information seems to be more robustly linked to pediatric asthma outcomes of interest.

Allergy describes a constellation of clinical diseases that affect up to 30% of the world's population. It is characterized by production of allergen-specific IgE, which binds to mast cells and initiates a cascade of molecular and cellular events that affect the respiratory tract (rhinitis and asthma), skin (dermatitis, urticaria), and multiple systems (anaphylaxis) in response to a variety of allergens including pollens, mold spores, animal danders, insect stings, foods, and drugs. The underlying pathophysiology involves immunoregulatory dysfunctions similar to those noted in highly stressed populations. The relationships in terms of potential for intervention are discussed.

The stress response influences the immune system, and studies in laboratory animals indicate that the response to stress significantly reduces resistance to infectious challenge. Only a few studies, however, have determined the impact of the stress response on human susceptibility to infectious challenge due, in part, to the difficulties of using live, replicating pathogens in human research. As a result, many studies have assessed the immune response to vaccination as a surrogate for the immune response to an infectious challenge. Thus, much is known about how the stress response influences adaptive immunity, and memory responses, to vaccination. These studies have yielded data concerning the interactions of the nervous and immune systems and have provided important information for clinicians administering vaccines to susceptible populations. This review provides a brief overview of the immune response to commonly used vaccines and the impact that stress can have on vaccine-specific immunity.

Converging and replicated evidence indicates that psychological stress can modulate wound-healing processes. This article reviews the methods and findings of experimental models of wound healing. Psychological stress can have a substantial and clinically relevant impact on wound repair. Physiologic stress responses can directly influence wound-healing processes. Furthermore, psychological stress can indirectly modulate the repair process by promoting the adoption of health-damaging behaviors. Translational work is needed to develop innovative treatments able to attenuate stress-induced delays in wound healing.

Age-related changes in immune function leave older adults at risk for a host of inflammatory diseases. Immune-mediated inflammatory processes are regulated by neuroendocrine hormones, including glucocorticoids, dehydroepiandrosterone, and the catecholamines, epinephrine, and norepinephrine. This regulation, however, becomes impaired in older adults in light of age-related changes in endocrine function. Chronic stress shows similarly harmful effects on neuroendocrine and immune function and may, therefore, combine with age to further increase disease risk in older adults. This article highlights evidence for the impact of age and stress on neuroendocrine regulation of inflammatory processes that may substantially increase risk for inflammatory disease at older ages.

This review focuses on the contributions of stress-related behavioral factors to cancer growth and metastasis and the biobehavioral mechanisms underlying these relationships. Behavioral factors that are important in modulation of the stress response and the pivotal role of neuroendocrine regulation in the downstream alteration of physiologic pathways relevant to cancer control, including the cellular immune response, inflammation, and tumor angiogenesis, invasion, and cell signaling pathways are described. Consequences for cancer progression and metastasis, as well as quality of life, are delineated. Behavioral and pharmacologic interventions with the potential to alter these biobehavioral pathways for patients with cancer are discussed.

Psychological stress has known effects on the immune system, including impacting effector and regulatory components. This can result in increased susceptibility to various infections, latent virus reactivation, and impact on immunoregulatory circuits. One of the great challenges in translational research is defining the risks associated with stress in specific patient populations and individuals. Future studies must include identification and validation of biomarkers that can categorize patient risk for adverse immune effects from various forms and degrees of psychological stress and how this impacts the course of their inflammatory disease.

THE CLINICS ARE NOW AVAILABLE ONLINE!
Access your subscription at:
www.theclinics.com

Foreword
The Stress of Writing
About Stress

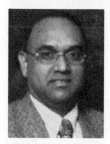

Rafeul Alam, MD, PhD
Consulting Editor

I want to write this foreword by describing my own state of the mind when approaching to write it. First, there is this deadline to meet, which is a stress for the mind. There is subconscious worry that I may forget it or miss the deadline. When I sit down to write it, I recognize that I have to write about a subject which is not my field of expertise. So, I do not feel sure about what to write. I could read up and then write, but will it make a difference? There is concern about how it will be perceived. You are now beginning to see what we all go through in dealing with matters in our daily life. Once we have dealt with the matter, we feel more relaxed when dealing with it for the second time. This is adaptation, which is the most important factor that determines the outcome of stress. Some of us are more adaptive, so we do not develop any negative consequences of stress. Those of us who are less adaptive fall victim to the stress. The adaptation to stress lies at the root of biological evolution. Biological processes are continuously evolving to adapt to the changing hostile environment and to reduce stress to the system. This ability to adapt is the fundamental feature of higher organisms and is also linked to longevity of the lifespan of a given species or individual. The complexity of the immune system, the hypothalamus-pituitary-adrenal axis, and the formation of novel hippocampal circuitry in response to stress[1] in higher organisms attests to this adaptiveness. The stress response at the individual cell level is better understood thanks to the development of modern biochemical and genetic tools. The response seems to follow the classic paradigm of Seyle's general adaptation syndrome. A single challenge with a stressor induces robust genomic changes in the cell, whereas repetitive challenge leads to adaptation and tolerance development

This work was supported by NIH Grants RO1 AI059719 and AI68088, PPG HL 36577, and N01 HHSN272200700048C.

Immunol Allergy Clin N Am 31 (2011) xi–xii
doi:10.1016/j.iac.2010.10.002
0889-8561/11/$ – see front matter © 2011 Elsevier Inc. All rights reserved.

immunology.theclinics.com

at the gene level.[2] Further, repetitive challenge leads to an alteration in system behavior. For example, the system develops signaling bistability, which is a biochemical process that may serve as memory.

The stress response at the level of the whole organism is far more complex and poorly understood. Many of our patients claim that their disease was either triggered or exacerbated by a stress. Many of us believe in this testimony but we are unable to test for it due to the inadequate knowledge about stress-related biochemical markers. Progress has been made in this very challenging field of medicine. Dr Gailen Marshall, who himself is a stress-scientist and a strong enthusiast of the field, has invited a group of devoted scientists to update us on the progress in the field. Hopefully, your stress will be less after reading this issue.

Rafeul Alam, MD, PhD
Division of Allergy and Immunology
National Jewish Health and
University of Colorado Denver Health Sciences Center
1400 Jackson Street
Denver, CO 80206, USA

E-mail address:
alamr@njc.org

REFERENCES

1. Lyons DM, Buckmaster PS, Lee AG, et al. Stress coping stimulates hippocampal neurogenesis in adult monkeys. Proc Natl Acad Sci U S A 2010;107:14823–7.
2. Liu W, Tundwal K, Liang Q, et al. Establishment of extracellular signal-regulated kinase 1/2 bistability and sustained activation through Sprouty 2 and its relevance for epithelial function. Mol Cell Biol 2010;30:1783–99.

Preface

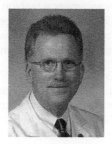

Gailen D. Marshall Jr, MD, PhD
Guest Editor

This issue of *Immunology and Allergy Clinics of North America* is, in some ways, a translational follow-up to a previous issue on psychoneuroimmunology. The principles laid down in that volume are the basis for the description of the effects of psychological stress on several clinical manifestations of inflammation. We have attempted to provide broad clinical examples of the proposed immune effects that are common to all inflammatory diseases as well as specific pathways unique to particular inflammatory diseases.

It is well appreciated by clinicians that patients who experience severe and/or chronic stressful situations have more complicated outcomes than those who do not. Further, those equipped with coping styles such as optimistic outlook, support systems, and well-developed belief systems tend to have better clinical outcomes. These clinical models (and some well-developed animal models) allow the examination of specific immunoregulatory and effector mechanisms in the patient populations that are already affected by an excess or deficiency of inflammatory pathways. Understanding these mechanisms will allow a more targeted approach to therapy that involves accounting for these stress-induced immune changes.

This volume is written by both established senior experts in the field and some exciting young investigators who will be the future leaders in PNI research. These articles describe work involving stress and aging, allergy, asthma, autoimmunity, malignancy, vaccine responses, and wound healing. The volume provides an excellent overview of the field with application for clinicians and researchers alike. The articles are organized to provide a statement of the clinical problem that involves stress and inflammatory diseases, and a description of work that has been done to address the mechanisms that may be involved in if not completely responsible for the adverse clinical outcomes. The clinical spectrum varies from an essentially deregulated system (ie, autoimmunity, allergy, asthma) to an overregulated/deficient immune system (ie, altered wound healing, impaired vaccine responses, malignancy), all adversely affected by chronic stress. Proposed mechanisms as well as strategies to more personally identify the most stress-susceptible individuals are also discussed.

This volume is the culmination of the efforts of many people. I wish to thank each listed author for his/her expertise, time, and efforts to make each article an outstanding

Immunol Allergy Clin N Am 31 (2011) xiii–xiv
doi:10.1016/j.iac.2010.10.001   **immunology.theclinics.com**
0889-8561/11/$ – see front matter © 2011 Elsevier Inc. All rights reserved.

one. I also thank Dr Rafuel Alam for the opportunity to prepare and guest-edit this tome. Special thanks go to Patrick Manley of Elsevier Publishers for his editorial guidance and patience with us as we worked to complete this in as timely a fashion as possible. Finally, on behalf of my coauthors, special thanks to all our family members, friends, and colleagues for their support and indulgence of us as we took time to work on this project. I trust you, the reader, will find that all our efforts have been worthwhile.

Gailen D. Marshall Jr, MD, PhD
Laboratory of Behavioral Immunology Research
Division of Clinical Immunology and Allergy
Department of Medicine
The University of Mississippi Medical Center
2500 North State Street
Jackson, MS 39216-4505, USA

E-mail address:
gmarshall@umc.edu

Stress and Autoimmunity

Courtney J. McCray, MD, Sandeep K. Agarwal, MD, PhD*

KEYWORDS

• Rheumatoid arthritis • Stress • Autoimmunity
• Neuroendocrine system

A common observation by physicians is the adverse relationship between stress and disease in patients. The association of stress and disease has been particularly true in regard to immune-based diseases, including susceptibility to infection, atopic diseases, and asthma. In addition, there has long been an interest in the relationship between stress and autoimmune diseases. Autoimmunity results from a dysregulated immune response against self.[1] Under normal physiologic conditions autoimmunity may be a phenomenological event without pathologic implications (eg, false positive autoantibody tests). Clinical autoimmune diseases occur when the autoimmune reaction results in tissue damage and destruction. Given the ability of stress and its downstream neuroendocrine alterations to modulate immune function,[2] it is reasonable to hypothesize that stress may influence autoimmunity and autoimmune disease. Although studies are conflicting, links between stress and autoimmune and inflammatory diseases, such as rheumatoid arthritis (RA), juvenile RA, systemic lupus erythematosus, and ankylosing spondylitis, likely exists.[3–6] Understanding the role that stress may have in either precipitating these diseases or triggering flare in the activity of these diseases could have implications for the treating physicians and patients. Translation of these findings into potential therapeutic interventions may provide a relatively safe and low-cost complement to traditional therapies in the management of these diseases.

Although stress likely has an impact on multiple autoimmune diseases, in the current article, the focus is on RA, using it as a model for stress-autoimmune interactions. The evidence that either supports or contradicts the potential role of stress in triggering autoimmune disease is discussed. Also, the evidence that supports stress as an important factor that may modify disease activity in RA patients is reviewed. Finally, the potential interventions aimed at stress that may one day become part of the therapeutic regimen in RA patients are discussed.

Division of Rheumatology and Clinical Immunogenetics, Department of Internal Medicine, University of Texas Health Science Center at Houston (UTHSC-H), 6431 Fannin Street, MSB 5.278, Houston, TX 77030, USA
* Corresponding author.
E-mail address: Sandeep.K.Agarwal@uth.tmc.edu

Immunol Allergy Clin N Am 31 (2011) 1–18
doi:10.1016/j.iac.2010.09.004
0889-8561/11/$ – see front matter. Published by Elsevier Inc.

RA

RA is a chronic, systemic autoimmune disease that primarily targets the synovial membrane of diarthrodial joints.[7] RA affects approximately 1% of the population, and is most common in patients 40 to 70 years old, but can affect patients at any age. Untreated, RA leads to joint damage and destruction, resulting in profound disability and loss of productivity at a substantial societal cost, as well as an increase in mortality. Fortunately, disease modifying therapies exist. Treatment with metho-trexate and other synthetic disease modifying agents clearly improves outcomes in patients with RA.[8] A substantial number of patients require treatment with biologics targeting cytokines (tumor necrosis factor-α [TNF-α], interleukin [IL]-1, IL-6), B cells, and T cell costimulation.[8]

A detailed review of the pathogenesis is beyond the scope of this article and can be found in several recent articles.[7,8] However, it is important to recognize that the path-ogenesis of RA involves a complex interaction of cells of the innate (neutrophils, mast cells, dendritic cells) and adaptive (T cells, B cells) immune systems. Furthermore, it is clear that a cytokine network, including TNF-α, IL-1, and IL-6, is central to the devel-opment of the inflammatory response in RA. It is not currently known what triggers the development of RA, nor is it understood what factors trigger flares in disease activity. Therefore, understanding additional modifiable factors that modulate susceptibility or activity of RA is of interest.

Is Stress a Trigger for Development of RA?

Although our understanding of the autoimmune and inflammatory pathways involved in the pathogenesis of RA continues to grow, the initial trigger for the development of RA remains elusive. Current paradigms implicate an aberrant immune response in a genetically predisposed individual to an environmental trigger that has yet be deter-mined.[1] However, these paradigms do not adequately explain why a genetically pre-disposed individual might develop an autoimmune disease at a specific point in time.

Indeed, it has long been suggested that psychological stress may be a trigger of RA. In 1942, a retrospective study of 20 RA patients reported that nearly half of the subjects attributed the onset of symptoms with a discrete, emotionally upsetting event.[9] In a subsequent editorial, it was noted that among 43 patients with RA, a significant number of patients mentioned the loss of social support (ie, loss of a spouse) coincident with onset of RA symptoms.[10,11] These findings were also confirmed in a retrospective study of 30 RA patients compared with 25 osteoarthritis (OA) patients.[10,11] Finally, a retrospective study of 100 women with RA, suggested that there were two distinct groups of RA patients: a major conflict group whose onset of symptoms occurred within a year of a traumatic life event and a nonconflict group whose disease onset was not associated with a preceding emotional event.[12] Interestingly, the major conflict group had an abrupt disease onset and a more severe disease course while the nonconflict group had a more insidious disease onset and a less severe disease course. Unfortunately, these studies do not provide details with regard to the diagnosis of RA, and some predate the use of diagnostic laboratories, radiological methods, and criteria that form a well-established definition of the diagnosis of RA. However, these studies are among the initial observations that formed the foundation for the hypothesis that psychological stress may be a trigger for the development of RA.

Several retrospective studies have further supported the association of stress preceding RA onset and have used diagnostic criteria for RA.[13,14] A retrospective study by Stewart and colleagues[15] also confirmed the prior observation that two subgroups of RA patients exist based on a different reactivity to stress.[12] In this study, 53 women with RA who met American College of Rheumatology (ACR) Criteria for the diagnosis of RA[16] were included, and rheumatoid factor (RF) status was determined for each subject. Interviews included measurement of pain, functional status, life events over past 10 years, and disease onset. Interestingly, the seronegative subgroup (negative RF) reported significantly higher rate of negative life events in the two years before disease onset.

Whereas several small retrospective studies have supported the association of stress with the onset of RA, there are also several studies that have failed to confirm this association. A large retrospective case-control study of 532 subjects failed to show a significant association in the occurrence of stressful events before onset of RA.[17] More recently, a prospective cohort of 9,159 subjects also failed to show a significant increased risk of developing RA in subjects reporting traumatic childhood experiences.[18] Although the size of the subject populations in these studies is a strength, neither study used rigid diagnostic criteria for the diagnosis of RA. Two additional studies have failed to confirm the hypothesis that stress may be a trigger for the development of RA. In a retrospective study of 60 subjects with ACR-classified RA, no significant association with stressful events preceding onset of disease in either seropositive or seronegative RA could be determined.[19] Finally, using a retrospective case-control study in which 55 subjects with RA-fulfilling ACR criteria were each matched with three controls, Carette and colleagues[20] failed to show a significant impact of stressful life events before the development of RA.

Based on the literature to date, the evidence for stress as a trigger for the development of RA remains controversial. The majority of studies supporting the idea of stress as a provoking factor in RA lack the statistical power to determine significance and their retrospective design is not ideal for determining causality. The two largest studies, including one that is prospective, found no significant association with stress and RA—thus favoring a lack of association.[17,18] However, failure to clearly see a consistent association may not rule out this possibility. The pathogenesis of RA is complex, and the ability to determine the timing of disease onset is often difficult. It is not clear if patients may have evidence of autoimmunity, for example the presence of anticyclic citrullinated peptide antibodies years before the development of clinical disease. Furthermore, the onset of RA in many patients is often insidious, with patients presenting to physicians only after symptoms reach an individual threshold. Indeed, Rimon[12] was able to show an association of stress in a group of patients with abrupt onset of RA but not in those with an insidious onset. It remains unclear if this reflects the variability of the disease, the difficulty of identifying disease onset, or the complexity of assessing stress and life events retrospectively. Future studies, ideally longitudinal studies, using diagnostic criteria and laboratory data may help resolve these controversies.

Does Stress Modulate Disease Activity in RA Patients?

Anecdotally, most physicians caring for patients with RA have observed that patients have increased symptoms during times of stress. Indeed, patients also have reported an association of psychological stress with RA symptoms. In a study of 92 RA patients, psychological stress was found to be the most common self-reported reason for disease flares.[21] The association of stress and RA flares has been a subject of investigation. Research has often divided stressful events, or stressors, into major and minor stressors. Major stressors are often life events such as death of a relative, severe illness of a relative, or separation from a partner. Minor stressors are often considered day-to-day events that an individual perceives as irritating or stressful. It is important to consider that a stress-associated increase in symptoms may be due to changes in pain or perception in pain. However, given the influence of stress on immune function, it is also possible that stress may have an impact on the inflammatory pathways that lead to increase synovial inflammation, thereby increasing a patient's symptoms. In this section the authors review the literature to address the question of whether major stressors or minor stressors modulate symptoms in RA patients.

Major stressors

It has been hypothesized that major stressors such as death of loved ones, natural disasters, or divorce can modulate disease activity with studies showing both a suppressive role and an exacerbating role. A case report of a woman with RA reported disease remission after death of her husband and daughter.[22] This report prompted a further study of 25 RA patients, of whom 6 had experienced death of a family member in the previous 6 months.[22] Joint tenderness was significantly lower for the bereaved group suggesting that major stressors may exert an immunosuppressive effect in RA patients.

In contrast, several studies have demonstrated that major stressors may be associated with a flare in RA activity. In a prospective study of 78 subjects with RA, those who experienced major life stressors in the preceding 6 months showed significantly increased pain with daily minor stressors.[23] Additionally, in a 15 year follow-up study of Rimon's[12] original study, the major conflict group whose disease onset was associated with traumatic life events later had significantly higher incidence of disease exacerbations with similar stressful events.[24] These studies support the hypothesis that major stressors are associated with an increase in RA symptoms.

Several studies have not shown association with major life events and RA disease activity. In a 5-year prospective study of 78 recently diagnosed RA patients, there was no significant relationship between major life stressors and disease activity, as measured by erythrocyte sedimentation rate (ESR) and a disease activity score.[25] However, disease activity was predicted by coping and social support at the time of diagnosis. In a multicenter prospective cohort study of 370 RA subjects meeting ACR criteria for RA, yearly interviews over the course of 3 years showed no significant association with major life events and disease activity, as determined by Ritchie Index, Health Assessment Questionnaire (HAQ), and Visual Analog Scale (VAS).[26] A 2-year prospective study of 238 RA patients meeting ACR criteria for RA showed no significant relationship between negative life events and worsened functional disability measured by the HAQ.[27] Additionally, studies by Dekkers and colleagues[28] and Thomason and colleagues[29] found no significant correlation between major life events and disease activity as measured by ESR.

Although data remains conflicting, at this time it appears that major stressors are not significantly associated with RA disease activity at the population level. The studies that demonstrate an association of major stressors with RA symptoms use pain as the outcome, whereas those that do not show the effect use measures that might better reflect inflammation. Could pain and inflammation in RA be differentially affected by major stressors? Additional studies using several standardized clinical diseases activity scales that have more recently been developed may be able to answer this question. Prospective studies performed with larger RA cohorts using either patient-driven disease activity scales such as the RA Disease Activity Index (RADAI) or the Clinical Disease Activity Index (CDAI), or multidimensional scales that combine physician measures, patient report, and laboratory markers, such as the disease activity score-28 (DAS28) or simplified disease activity index (SDAI), would permit more sensitive assessment of disease activity and help to demonstrate an association of major stressors and RA activity.[30]

Minor stressors

The majority of studies investigating the association of stress and RA-disease activity have focused on minor stressors, are hassles encountered on a daily basis, including interpersonal relations, work stress, and financial stressors. The majority of these studies have consistently demonstrated an association of increased RA symptoms with minor stressors. A 12-week prospective study of 41 women with RA diagnosed based on ACR criteria found a significant relationship between minor stressors and joint tenderness and pain.[31] Additionally, in a subgroup of 20 patients who experienced a highly stressful week during the study, significant increases in clinician global ratings of disease activity were associated with an increase in numbers of DR+ CD3 cells and IL-2 receptor were seen, which supports the hypothesis that minor stressors are associated with increased disease activity.[31] In the previously mentioned study by Potter and Zautra,[22] patients found daily stressors and negative affect significantly correlated with increased joint tenderness. Further supporting the association of minor stressors with RA activity is a 5-year prospective study of 50 RA patients. The investigators observed that patients with higher levels of daily stress had more joint swelling and erosions at study entry, and progression of these erosions continued over the course of the study.[32] Finally, interpersonal workplace stressors and financial stress have also been evaluated and found to significantly predict arthritis symptoms, including pain, as well as nonarthritis health complaints in both RA and OA patients.[33,34]

The role of mood disturbances in the stress-disease activity paradigm has also been evaluated. From a cohort of 138 RA patients, 74 patients were randomly assigned to undergo a controlled stress induction. Interestingly, those patients with history of two or more episodes of major depression had significantly increased pain as measured by Short Form-36 (SF-36), Western Ontario and McMaster Osteoarthritis Index (WOMAC), and DAS28 measure of tenderness.[3] Similarly, in another study of 14 RA patients, it was found that increases in joint inflammation were significantly correlated with increased soluble interleukin-2 receptor (sIL-2R) levels and increases in mood disturbance significantly correlated with declining sIL-2R levels and increased pain, suggesting that mood disturbances contribute to pain perceptions despite levels of underlying inflammation.[35] Similarly, increased daily stressors were associated with increased pain but decreased joint inflammation evidenced by diminished IL-2R, suggesting a role for mood disturbance in pain perception.[36] Collectively, the above studies suggest depression and other mood disturbances could increase vulnerability of RA patients to stress, thus accounting for differences in pain experienced by each person.

Only a few published studies have not shown an association with minor stressors and disease activity. In the study by Dekkers and colleagues,[28] 54 patients with newly diagnosed RA completed the Life Experience Survey, were assessed for coping skills and social support, as well as health status measures where evaluation included ESR and VAS. No significant correlation was observed between minor stressors and ESR or pain. A retrospective study of 66 RA patients found no significant correlation with psychosocial stress and pain; other disease activity markers were not evaluated.[37]

Taken together, the weight of the published evidence supports the association of minor stressors and RA disease activity. However, from these studies, it is not always clear if the increase in RA disease activity is immune mediated and through increased synovial inflammation, through changes in pain and pain perception, or both. The majority of studies cite pain as the most common measure of disease activity. Regardless of the mechanism, pain remains an important target in therapeutic intervention as it can significantly influence quality of life in RA patients. Undoubtedly, the relationship between stress and rheumatic disease is complex, and the mechanism of influence has not been elucidated through the studies available at this time.

Mechanisms of Stress-Associated RA Flares

As discussed above, minor stressors appear to be associated with increase symptoms in RA patients. The studies do not clearly distinguish if these symptoms are secondary to increases in inflammation and synovitis or alterations in pain. A thorough discussion of how stress can affect pain is beyond the scope of this article. However, it is important for the reader to appreciate the possibility that some of the stress-associated increase in symptoms in RA patients may be related to the effects of stress on pain pathways.[38] An alternative mechanism by which stress may increase symptoms in RA patients is through modulation of the immune response. Indeed, animal and human studies have demonstrated bidirectional communication of the neuroendocrine system and the immune system and have provided a conceptual framework for how stress may contribute to the pathogenesis of immune-mediated disease. This section discusses possible basic immune mechanisms by which stress may adversely affect symptoms or disease activity in RA patients.

Stress-immune interactions

The impact of stress on immune function has been extensively investigated using subjects with exposure to stressors such as bereavement, marital discord, caregiving for a relative with a chronic illness, and academic examination stress. Initial paradigms supported a potential suppressive effect of stress on immune function, including suppression of natural killer cell function, lymphocyte proliferation, and peripheral blood mononuclear cell (PBMC) production of IL-2 and interferon gamma (IFN-γ).[39–44] However, these experimental observations were inadequate to explain the association of stress with increased susceptibility to asthma and atopic diseases, immune-based diseases where T helper (Th)-2 cytokines are increased. Subsequent studies using the medical student examination stress model suggested that stress is associated with a shift in the Th-1 (type-1)/Th-2 (type-2) cytokine balance toward Th-2 cytokine responses.[45] These studies were confirmed with multiple in vitro studies where dexamethasone, at concentrations mimicking serum cortisol levels during periods of stress, suppressed IFN-γ production and increased the production of IL-4 and IL-10 by human PBMC, a shift toward a Th-2 cytokine milieu.[46,47] More recently, it has been demonstrated that exposure of corticosteroids can increase the sensitivity of PBMC to the immunomodulatory effects of catecholamines, providing evidence for a cooperative effect of multiple stress hormones in regulating Th-1 and Th-2 cytokines.[48] These data strongly suggested that stress is not immune suppressive, rather it modulates immune function such that it decreases Th-1 responses while increasing Th-2 responses.

After the identification of the Th-1 or Th-2 cytokine balance, a significant amount of research sought to explain the pathogenesis of autoimmune diseases using the imbalance of these two Th subsets. Initial studies suggested that Th-1 cytokines would support autoimmunity; however, several studies conflicted these data.[49] Subsequent studies demonstrated that a third Th subset, the Th-17 cell, may more adequately explain the CD4+ T cell contribution to autoimmune diseases.[50,51] Th-17 cells differentiate from naive Th cells when stimulated in the presence of IL-6, transforming growth factor-β, and IL-1β. IL-23 is another key cytokine that supports the Th-17 cytokine response. Indeed, several studies now support a potential role for Th-17 cells in autoimmune diseases, including RA.[52–54] Currently, no published studies have shown an association of stress with alterations in IL-17 or IL-23. However, an intriguing in vitro study using T cells from DO11.10 ova-specific transgenic mice demonstrated that dexamethasone did not decrease IL-17 and IL-22 production by Th-17 cells.[55] Although this study did not use "stress" equivalents of dexamethasone, these data, in combination with prior data demonstrating a decrease in Th-1 cytokines, suggest that corticosteroids and, possibly, stress may support a Th-17 milieu.

Regulatory T cells (T-reg) are a CD4+ T cell population that suppress immune responses through a variety of mechanisms.[56] Loss of T-reg function may contribute to autoimmunity and autoimmune disease.[56] It is of interest to understand whether stress may alter T-reg function, which in turn could modulate the immune balance and contribute to autoimmunity. Consistent with this hypothesis, patients with post-traumatic stress disorder have been found to have lower circulating T reg cells, as defined by intracellular expression of the T-reg transcription factor FoxP3, relative to age and ethnically matched controls.[57]

The therapeutic success of biologics targeting inflammatory cytokines such as TNF-α, IL-1β, and IL-6 highlight the important role that these cytokines play in the pathogenesis of RA.[58–61] The ability of stress to modulate the inflammatory cytokines represents another potential mechanism by which stressors may increased RA activity. One recent study examined circulating IL-6 levels in a large cohort of spousal dementia caregivers compared with controls.[62] Over the 6-year period, the average rate of increase in IL-6 levels in caregivers was approximately four times that of control subjects. Several studies also have demonstrated an association of increased IL-6 levels in RA patients with stress.[63–65] Another study demonstrated that a laboratory acute stressor resulted in higher levels of circulating IL-1β compared with controls.[66] Finally, a meta-analysis of 30 studies demonstrated robust effects for an increase in IL-6 and IL-1β following acute stress.[67] Together these studies suggest that stress is associated with an increase in proinflammatory cytokines, which may in part contribute to an increase in inflammation in RA patients owing to an increase in stressors.

One additional mechanism by which stress may affect RA is through regulation of telomerase and telomere length in T cells. It has been reported that CD4+ T cells from RA patients have accelerated telomere attrition.[68] This may be due to a defect in the upregulation of telomerase in RA patients, and this has been hypothesized to contribute to a defect in regulation of the T cell pool through excessive T cell loss. Interestingly, a recent study has reported an association of chronic caregiver stress with shorter telomere lengths in PBMC compared with controls.[69] Therefore, stress could potentially add to the telomere attrition in T cells, which may have an impact on the immune balance and inflammatory status in RA patients.

In summary, stress can modulate the immune response at multiple levels. Stress-induced alterations in Th cell subsets, T-regs, as well as inflammatory cytokines can have significant impact on the immune balance in healthy subjects. Similar changes have been seen in RA patients. Given the association of minor stressors with increased symptoms in RA patients, these stress-associated alterations likely contribute to a proinflammatory milieu in RA patients.

STRESS INTERVENTIONS IN RA MANAGEMENT

Given the potential association of minor stressors with RA flares and disease activity, it is important to understand if stress interventions could play a role in the management of RA. Although it is unlikely that stress management alone would induce remission in patients, combining stress intervention with pharmacologic intervention may be an effective way to reduce the need for some medications, such as corticosteroids. This would reduce treatment side effects and offer patients safe and complementary interventions in the management of their disease. A large number of studies have sought to determine if stress interventions are safe and beneficial in the management of RA, including a large number of randomized controlled trials summarized in **Table 1**. This section reviews the published studies investigating psychological interventions such as cognitive behavioral therapy and emotional disclosure, as well as other methodologies that indirectly modulate stress levels such as tai chi, yoga, and patient education.

Psychological Interventions

Cognitive behavioral therapy

Many studies on cognitive behavior therapy (CBT) for treatment of RA have been conducted and involve therapist-guided training in coping strategies such as relaxation, goal setting, imagery, and cognitive restructuring of negative thoughts related to pain.[70] In a randomized controlled trial of 53 RA patients, each were assigned to the CBT group, social support therapy group, or a nontreatment group. Significant improvements in disease activity as measured by Rheumatoid Activity Index, pain, pain behavior, and anxiety were seen posttreatment and at 6 month follow-up.[71] Sharpe and colleagues[72] conducted a randomized clinical trial of 54 RA patients comparing routine medical care with or without CBT. CBT resulted in significant improvements in joint stiffness, depression, and C-reactive protein (CRP) posttreatment, as well as joint stiffness and depression at 6-month follow-up. At 18 months, patients maintained initial treatment gains with additional significant improvement in anxiety and disability.[73]

In contrast to the above positive studies, other studies have shown no effect on disease activity. In a randomized controlled trial of 63 RA patients, the experimental group received weekly CBT sessions with significant improvements in pain coping, depression, affective pain score, and emotional stabilization.[74] However, no significant effect on disease activity as measured by ESR, CRP, and joint counts was observed.[74] CBT resulted in significant improvement in depression and fatigue but not disease activity in a randomized controlled trial involving individualized CBT in 64 RA patients.[75] Similarly, studies by Parker and colleagues[76,77] and O'Leary and colleagues[78] showed significant improvement in pain, pain coping, and self efficacy with CBT, but no effects on disease activity as measured by ESR, CRP, Th subsets, and joint counts. The above studies provide evidence that CBT is an effective therapeutic intervention in RA, especially in the areas of pain, pain coping, self-efficacy, and depression. Effects on disease activity and disability are seen in some studies suggesting a potential role; however, more studies are needed to clarify this effect.

Emotional disclosure

Emotional disclosure is a therapeutic modality in which patients write or talk about their thoughts and feelings concerning life events that are not yet disclosed to others. It has been suggested that emotional disclosure has health benefits, thus a few studies have evaluated its role in treatment of RA.[79] In a randomized controlled trial of 72 RA patients in which the experimental group was assigned to talk about stressful events and the control group about trivial topics, significant improvement in affective and physical functioning was seen with no effect on pain or joint counts.[80] Another randomized controlled trial of 51 RA patients found significant improvement in disease activity as measured by physician global assessment 4 months after treatment.[81] Significant improvement in mood indices but not disease activity was seen in a randomized controlled trial of 34 RA patients who were assigned to write and talk about traumatic personal experiences.[82] In contrast, Keefe and colleagues[83] found no significant benefit of clinician assisted emotional disclosure on pain, disability, or affect. Given as there have been very few published studies on the effect of emotional disclosure on RA disease activity, no conclusions can be made at this time. Though it appears there could be beneficial effects on mood indices and potentially on disease activity, more studies are needed to further delineate the role of emotional disclosure in RA therapy.

Tai Chi

Tai chi is a traditional Chinese martial art that combines slow and graceful movements with mental focus. It has been found to provide benefit to cardiopulmonary function, strength, balance, flexibility, and psychological function.[84] Additionally, it has also been hypothesized to be a therapeutic option in RA. A systematic review including studies by Kirsteins and colleagues[85] and Van Deusen and Harlowe[86] concluded that tai chi provides significant improvement in lower extremity range of motion with no other significant beneficial or detrimental effects on disease activity.[87] Subsequently, several studies have shown therapeutic benefit of tai chi in RA. In a randomized controlled trial of 20 RA patients, the experimental group performed tai chi twice weekly for 12 weeks while the control group underwent RA education along with stretching exercises. Results showed significant improvement in disability index, quality of life, and depression index.[88] Uhlig and colleagues[89] conducted a single group clinical study in which 15 RA patients performed tai chi twice weekly for 12 weeks and underwent baseline, posttreatment, and 12-week follow-up assessments of joint tenderness (DAS28), physical performance tests, functional disability (HAQ), and pain (VAS). Significant improvements in the number of swollen joints, lower limb strength, and endurance was seen at the end of study and follow up, and patients reported increased confidence in movement as well as overall reduced pain. These findings are contradictory to an earlier, similar study that reported no significant improvement in the same measures.[90] The few studies that have been conducted are small, thus improvement in strength of the studies and possibly increased effect could be seen if larger sample sizes were used. Overall, it can be concluded that tai chi can be safely performed without causing exacerbation of disease with evidence for improved lower extremity strength, flexibility, and endurance. It is likely that quality of life and functional disability could be improved with continued tai chi practice as well.

Yoga

Yoga has been found to have positive mood and fitness effects.[91,92] However, few studies have been conducted to evaluate the effect of yoga on RA disease activity. In a clinical controlled trial of 47 RA patients, the experimental group participated in an 8-week yoga program and showed significant improvements in disease activity (DAS28) and disability (HAQ).[93] Another study of 16 women with RA who practiced yoga for 10 weeks found significant improvements HAQ, perception of pain and depression, as well as improved balance compared with the control group.[94] Studies by Haslock and colleagues[95] and Dash and Telles[96] showed improvement in grip strength after practicing yoga. At this time, no conclusions can be made regarding the effects of yoga on RA disease activity given the paucity of published studies. Beneficial effects of yoga on flexibility, endurance, and mood have been demonstrated in individuals without RA, so it is probable these same effects could be seen RA patients.

Table 1
Randomized controlled trials for stress interventions in the management of RA

First Author (Year)	Intervention	Sample Size	Results
Bradley (1987)[71]	CBT—5 individual thermal biofeedback sessions with 10 small group meetings	53	Postintervention and follow-up: significant improvement in pain, and RAI
Sharpe (2001)[72]	CBT—8 weekly sessions including relaxation, pain coping, education	53	Postintervention: significant improvement in joint stiffness, depression, CRP 6-mo follow-up: significant improvement depression and stiffness
Sharpe (2003)[73]	CBT—same as above	53	Maintained significant improvement in depression, joint stiffness Additional improvement in anxiety and disability
Lebing (1999)[74]	CBT—12 weekly sessions involving relaxation, pain management, coping	55	Significant improvements in pain coping, depression, affective pain score, and emotional stabilization
Evers (2002)[75]	CBT—10 biweekly individually tailored sessions	64	Significant improvement in depression and pain
Parker (1995)[76]	CBT—10 weekly stress management sessions with 15 mo maintenance program	141	Significant improvement in helplessness, self-efficacy, coping at 15 mo follow up.
Parker (1988)[77]	CBT—1 wk inpatient program with 6 group maintenance sessions involving coping	83	Significant improvement in pain, coping postintervention and 6 and 12 mo follow-up
O'Leary (1988)[78]	CBT—5 weekly sessions including relaxation, attention refocusing, self-encouragement	33	Significant improvement in self efficacy and coping at 4 mo
Kelley (1997)[80]	Emotional Disclosure—verbal stressful events on 4 consecutive days	72	Significant improvement in affective disturbance and physical functioning at 3 mo
Smyth (1999)[81]	Emotional Disclosure—written disclosure of most stressful event	51	Significant improvement in disease activity at 4 mo
Wetherell (2005)[82]	Emotional Disclosure—written or verbal disclosure traumatic personal experiences on 4 consecutive days	34	Significant improvement in mood indices at 10 wk follow up

Keefe (2008)[83]	98	Emotional Disclosure—verbal disclosure about traumatic personal experiences privately or with clinician	No significant improvement in any measures
Han (2004)[87]	206	Tai chi—Various programs with tai chi instruction or philosophy	Significant improvement in ankle plantar flexion No detrimental effects
Wang (2008)[88]	20	Tai chi—Twice weekly sessions for 12 wk	Significant improvement in disability and depression
Lorig (1985)[98]	190 (11% RA)	Education—Arthritis Self Management Program; 6 sessions	Significant improvement in knowledge, behaviors (exercise, relaxation), and diminished pain at 4 mo and 20 mo
Lorig (1993)[99]	190	Education—4 y follow up study	Significant improvement in pain and decreased number of physician office visits
Barlow (2000)[100]	544 (70 RA)	Education—Arthritis Self Management Program; 6 weekly sessions	Significant improvement in cognitive symptoms management, mood, communication with physician and depression at 4 mo and 1 y Significant improvement in pain at 1 y
Lindroth (1997)[101]	100	Education—8 weekly sessions	Significant increased knowledge, exercise, joint protection, and signify significant decreased pain and disability at 3 mo Only increased knowledge and joint protection at 12 mo
Hill (2001)[103]	100	Education—7 sessions	Significant increased adherence in taking medication (D-penicillamine) at 24 mo
Riemsma (2003)[104]	Not given	Education—meta analysis of 31 RCTs	Significant improvement in disability, joint counts, patient global assessment, psychological status, and depression at first follow-up No significant effects seen at final follow up (3–12 m)

Abbreviations: RAI, rheumatoid activity index; RCTs, randomized controlled trials.

Education

Some of the earliest work in educational programs for treatment of RA was done by Lorig[97] through development of the Arthritis Self-Management Program. An early study found that the program resulted in significant improvement in knowledge, behaviors such as exercise and relaxation, as well as diminished pain.[98] A 4-year follow-up study showed long-term benefit as significant decreases in pain and physician visits were found.[99] A larger randomized controlled trial of 544 OA and RA patients found that those who completed the self-management program had significant improvement in cognitive symptoms, communication with physicians, and pain, as well as significant decrease in depression and visits to physicians at 1-year follow-up.[100] Although these studies were predominantly comprised of OA patients, other studies in RA patients have shown similar benefit. A controlled trial of 100 RA patients randomized to a problem-based education group and a control group found significant short-term increases in knowledge, exercise, and joint protection behaviors, as well as significant decreases in pain and disability. The only long-term effects seen were increased knowledge and joint protection.[101] A two-part study by Scholten and colleagues[102] found participation in an educational program resulted in significant postintervention improvement in coping strategies, depression, disability, and compliance with therapy; at 5-year follow-up, significant gains in disability, coping, and compliance were maintained. Likewise, similar improvement in treatment adherence was seen in a randomized controlled trial by Hill and colleagues.[103] A systematic review of 31 randomized controlled trials found significant short-term effects of education on disability, patient global assessment, and depression with no effect on disease activity. No significant long-term effects were seen.[104] The above studies demonstrate that educational interventions have significant short-term effects on disability, depression, pain, knowledge, and perhaps treatment adherence. Long-term benefit is uncertain at this time, warranting future follow-up studies to further evaluate the potential effect on disease activity.

SUMMARY

The importance of stress on immune function and balance has long been of interest, and our appreciation for the effects that stress can have on immune-based diseases continues to grow. Published studies do support the concept that stress can have a significant impact on autoimmune diseases, in particular rheumatoid arthritis. Whereas the effects of stress on onset of RA may be equivocal, the literature supports a role for minor stressors as factors that can contribute to symptom flares in RA patients. Furthermore, stress reduction interventions can have a positive therapeutic effect in RA patients as well. These are of particular interest given that a significant number of patients seek alternatives that can be combined with pharmacologic and biologic therapies to better manage their disease. A need persists to further investigate the effect of stress and stress interventions in RA using more sensitive tools that assess RA activity as well as measurements of stress. Until these studies emerge, it is important for physicians and patients to recognize the potential for stress to impact RA and autoimmune diseases and how stress management should be considered in a multidimensional approach to RA.

REFERENCES

1. Ermann J, Fathman CG. Autoimmune diseases: genes, bugs and failed regulation. Nat Immunol 2001;2(9):759–61.

2. Agarwal SK, Marshall GD Jr. Stress effects on immunity and its application to clinical immunology. Clin Exp Allergy 2001;31(1):25–31.
3. Zautra AJ, Parrish BP, Van Puymbroeck CM, et al. Depression history, stress, and pain in rheumatoid arthritis patients. J Behav Med 2007;30(3): 187–97.
4. Brionez TF, Assassi S, Reveille JD, et al. Psychological correlates of self-reported disease activity in ankylosing spondylitis. J Rheumatol 2010;37(4): 829–34.
5. Vandvik IH, Hoyeraal HM, Fagertun H. Chronic family difficulties and stressful life events in recent onset juvenile arthritis. J Rheumatol 1989;16(8):1088–92.
6. Pawlak CR, Witte T, Heiken H, et al. Flares in patients with systemic lupus erythematosus are associated with daily psychological stress. Psychother Psychosom 2003;72(3):159–65.
7. Lee DM, Weinblatt ME. Rheumatoid arthritis. Lancet 2001;358(9285):903–11.
8. O'Dell JR. Therapeutic strategies for rheumatoid arthritis. N Engl J Med 2004; 350(25):2591–602.
9. Halliday JL. Psychological aspects of rheumatoid arthritis. Proc R Soc Med 1942;35(7):455–7.
10. Robinson CE. Emotional factors and rheumatoid arthritis. Can Med Assoc J 1957;77(4):344–5.
11. Pancheri P, Teodori S, Aparo UL. Psychological aspects of rheumatoid arthritis vis-a-vis osteoarthrosis. Scand J Rheumatol 1978;7(1):42–8.
12. Rimon R. Social and psychosomatic aspects of rheumatoid arthritis. Acta Rheumatol Scand 1969;13(Suppl):1+.
13. Latman NS, Walls R. Personality and stress: an exploratory comparison of rheumatoid arthritis and osteoarthritis. Arch Phys Med Rehabil 1996;77(8): 796–800.
14. Marcenaro M, Prete C, Badini A, et al. Rheumatoid arthritis, personality, stress response style, and coping with illness. A preliminary survey. Ann N Y Acad Sci 1999;876:419–25.
15. Stewart MW, Knight RG, Palmer DG, et al. Differential relationships between stress and disease activity for immunologically distinct subgroups of people with rheumatoid arthritis. J Abnorm Psychol 1994;103(2):251–8.
16. Arnett FC, Edworthy SM, Bloch DA, et al. The American Rheumatism Association 1987 revised criteria for the classification of rheumatoid arthritis. Arthritis Rheum 1988;31(3):315–24.
17. EmpireRheumatismCouncil. A controlled investigation into the aetiology and clinical features of rheumatoid arthritis. BMJ 1950;1:799.
18. Kopec JA, Sayre EC. Traumatic experiences in childhood and the risk of arthritis: a prospective cohort study. Can J Public Health 2004;95(5):361–5.
19. Conway SC, Creed FH, Symmons DP. Life events and the onset of rheumatoid arthritis. J Psychosom Res 1994;38(8):837–47.
20. Carette S, Surtees PG, Wainwright NW, et al. The role of life events and childhood experiences in the development of rheumatoid arthritis. J Rheumatol 2000;27(9):2123–30.
21. Affleck G, Pfeiffer C, Tennen H, et al. Attributional processes in rheumatoid arthritis patients. Arthritis Rheum 1987;30(8):927–31.
22. Potter PT, Zautra AJ. Stressful life events' effects on rheumatoid arthritis disease activity. J Consult Clin Psychol 1997;65(2):319–23.
23. Affleck G, Tennen H, Urrows S, et al. Person and contextual features of daily stress reactivity: individual differences in relations of undesirable daily events

with mood disturbance and chronic pain intensity. J Pers Soc Psychol 1994; 66(2):329–40.

24. Rimon R, Laakso RL. Life stress and rheumatoid arthritis. A 15-year follow-up study. Psychother Psychosom 1985;43(1):38–43.

25. Evers AW, Kraaimaat FW, Geenen R, et al. Stress-vulnerability factors as long-term predictors of disease activity in early rheumatoid arthritis. J Psychosom Res 2003;55(4):293–302.

26. Leymarie F, Jolly D, Sanderman R, et al. Life events and disability in rheumatoid arthritis: a European cohort. Br J Rheumatol 1997;36(10):1106–12.

27. Smedstad LM, Kvien TK, Moum T, et al. Life events, psychosocial factors, and demographic variables in early rheumatoid arthritis: relations to one-year changes in functional disability. J Rheumatol 1995;22(12):2218–25.

28. Dekkers JC, Geenen R, Evers AW, et al. Biopsychosocial mediators and moderators of stress-health relationships in patients with recently diagnosed rheumatoid arthritis. Arthritis Rheum 2001;45(4):307–16.

29. Thomason BT, Brantley PJ, Jones GN, et al. The relation between stress and disease activity in rheumatoid arthritis. J Behav Med 1992;15(2):215–20.

30. Dougados M, Aletaha D, van Riel P. Disease activity measures for rheumatoid arthritis. Clin Exp Rheumatol 2007;25(5 Suppl 46):S22–9.

31. Zautra AJ, Hoffman J, Potter P, et al. Examination of changes in interpersonal stress as a factor in disease exacerbations among women with rheumatoid arthritis. Ann Behav Med 1997;19(3):279–86.

32. Feigenbaum SL, Masi AT, Kaplan SB. Prognosis in rheumatoid arthritis. A longitudinal study of newly diagnosed younger adult patients. Am J Med 1979;66(3):377–84.

33. Potter PT, Smith BW, Strobel KR, et al. Interpersonal workplace stressors and well-being: a multi-wave study of employees with and without arthritis. J Appl Psychol 2002;87(4):789–96.

34. Skinner MA, Zautra AJ, Reich JW. Financial stress predictors and the emotional and physical health of chronic pain patients. Cognit Ther Res 2004;28(5): 695–713.

35. Harrington L, Affleck G, Urrows S, et al. Temporal covariation of soluble interleukin-2 receptor levels, daily stress, and disease activity in rheumatoid arthritis. Arthritis Rheum 1993;36(2):199–203.

36. Affleck G, Urrows S, Tennen H, et al. A dual pathway model of daily stressor effects on rheumatoid arthritis. Ann Behav Med 1997;19(2):161–70.

37. Radanov BP, Frost SA, Schwarz HA, et al. Experience of pain in rheumatoid arthritis—an empirical evaluation of the contribution of developmental psychosocial stress. Acta Psychiatr Scand 1996;93(6):482–8.

38. Clauw DJ. Fibromyalgia: an overview. Am J Med 2009;122(Suppl 12):S3–13.

39. Schleifer SJ, Keller SE, Camerino M, et al. Suppression of lymphocyte stimulation following bereavement. JAMA 1983;250(3):374–7.

40. Kiecolt-Glaser JK, Garner W, Speicher C, et al. Psychosocial modifiers of immunocompetence in medical students. Psychosom Med 1984;46(1):7–14.

41. Kiecolt-Glaser JK, Glaser R, Strain EC, et al. Modulation of cellular immunity in medical students. J Behav Med 1986;9(1):5–21.

42. Glaser R, Pearson GR, Bonneau RH, et al. Stress and the memory T-cell response to the Epstein-Barr virus in healthy medical students. Health Psychol 1993;12(6):435–42.

43. Dobbin JP, Harth M, McCain GA, et al. Cytokine production and lymphocyte transformation during stress. Brain Behav Immun 1991;5(4):339–48.

44. Glaser R, Rice J, Sheridan J, et al. Stress-related immune suppression: health implications. Brain Behav Immun 1987;1(1):7–20.
45. Marshall GD Jr, Agarwal SK, Lloyd C, et al. Cytokine dysregulation associated with exam stress in healthy medical students. Brain Behav Immun 1998;12(4):297–307.
46. Agarwal SK, Marshall GD Jr. Glucocorticoid-induced type 1/type 2 cytokine alterations in humans: a model for stress-related immune dysfunction. J Interferon Cytokine Res 1998;18(12):1059–68.
47. Agarwal SK, Marshall GD Jr. Beta-adrenergic modulation of human type-1/type-2 cytokine balance. J Allergy Clin Immunol 2000;105(1 Pt 1):91–8.
48. Salicru AN, Sams CF, Marshall GD. Cooperative effects of corticosteroids and catecholamines upon immune deviation of the type-1/type-2 cytokine balance in favor of type-2 expression in human peripheral blood mononuclear cells. Brain Behav Immun 2007;21(7):913–20.
49. Cua DJ, Sherlock J, Chen Y, et al. Interleukin-23 rather than interleukin-12 is the critical cytokine for autoimmune inflammation of the brain. Nature 2003; 421(6924):744–8.
50. Bettelli E, Korn T, Kuchroo VK. Th17: the third member of the effector T cell trilogy. Curr Opin Immunol 2007;19(6):652–7.
51. Bettelli E, Oukka M, Kuchroo VK. T(H)-17 cells in the circle of immunity and autoimmunity. Nat Immunol 2007;8(4):345–50.
52. Amre DK, Mack D, Israel D, et al. Association between genetic variants in the IL-23R gene and early-onset Crohn's disease: results from a case-control and family-based study among Canadian children. Am J Gastroenterol 2008; 103(3):615–20.
53. Burton PR, Clayton DG, Cardon LR, et al. Association scan of 14,500 nonsynonymous SNPs in four diseases identifies autoimmunity variants. Nat Genet 2007; 39(11):1329–37.
54. Chu CQ, Swart D, Alcorn D, et al. Interferon-gamma regulates susceptibility to collagen-induced arthritis through suppression of interleukin-17. Arthritis Rheum 2007;56(4):1145–51.
55. McKinley L, Alcorn JF, Peterson A, et al. TH17 cells mediate steroid-resistant airway inflammation and airway hyperresponsiveness in mice. J Immunol 2008;181(6):4089–97.
56. Esensten JH, Wofsy D, Bluestone JA. Regulatory T cells as therapeutic targets in rheumatoid arthritis. Nat Rev Rheumatol 2009;5(10):560–5.
57. Sommershof A, Aichinger H, Engler H, et al. Substantial reduction of naive and regulatory T cells following traumatic stress. Brain Behav Immun 2009;23(8): 1117–24.
58. Choy EH, Panayi GS. Cytokine pathways and joint inflammation in rheumatoid arthritis. N Engl J Med 2001;344(12):907–16.
59. Weinblatt ME, Kremer JM, Bankhurst AD, et al. A trial of etanercept, a recombinant tumor necrosis factor receptor:Fc fusion protein, in patients with rheumatoid arthritis receiving methotrexate. N Engl J Med 1999;340(4):253–9.
60. Lipsky PE, van der Heijde DM, St Clair EW, et al. Infliximab and methotrexate in the treatment of rheumatoid arthritis. Anti-Tumor Necrosis Factor Trial in Rheumatoid Arthritis with Concomitant Therapy Study Group. N Engl J Med 2000; 343(22):1594–602.
61. Smolen JS, Beaulieu A, Rubbert-Roth A, et al. Effect of interleukin-6 receptor inhibition with tocilizumab in patients with rheumatoid arthritis (OPTION study): a double-blind, placebo-controlled, randomised trial. Lancet 2008;371(9617): 987–97.

62. Kiecolt-Glaser JK, Preacher KJ, MacCallum RC, et al. Chronic stress and age-related increases in the proinflammatory cytokine IL-6. Proc Natl Acad Sci U S A 2003;100(15):9090–5.
63. Zautra AJ, Yocum DC, Villanueva I, et al. Immune activation and depression in women with rheumatoid arthritis. J Rheumatol 2004;31(3):457–63.
64. Davis MC, Zautra AJ, Younger J, et al. Chronic stress and regulation of cellular markers of inflammation in rheumatoid arthritis: implications for fatigue. Brain Behav Immun 2008;22(1):24–32.
65. Hirano D, Nagashima M, Ogawa R, et al. Serum levels of interleukin 6 and stress related substances indicate mental stress condition in patients with rheumatoid arthritis. J Rheumatol 2001;28(3):490–5.
66. Yamakawa K, Matsunaga M, Isowa T, et al. Transient responses of inflammatory cytokines in acute stress. Biol Psychol 2009;82(1):25–32.
67. Steptoe A, Hamer M, Chida Y. The effects of acute psychological stress on circulating inflammatory factors in humans: a review and meta-analysis. Brain Behav Immun 2007;21(7):901–12.
68. Fujii H, Shao L, Colmegna I, et al. Telomerase insufficiency in rheumatoid arthritis. Proc Natl Acad Sci U S A 2009;106(11):4360–5.
69. Damjanovic AK, Yang Y, Glaser R, et al. Accelerated telomere erosion is associated with a declining immune function of caregivers of Alzheimer's disease patients. J Immunol 2007;179(6):4249–54.
70. Keefe FJ, Somers TJ, Martire LM. Psychologic interventions and lifestyle modifications for arthritis pain management. Rheum Dis Clin North Am 2008; 34(2):351–68.
71. Bradley LA, Young LD, Anderson KO, et al. Effects of psychological therapy on pain behavior of rheumatoid arthritis patients. Treatment outcome and six-month followup. Arthritis Rheum 1987;30(10):1105–14.
72. Sharpe L, Sensky T, Timberlake N, et al. A blind, randomized, controlled trial of cognitive-behavioural intervention for patients with recent onset rheumatoid arthritis: preventing psychological and physical morbidity. Pain 2001;89(2–3):275–83.
73. Sharpe L, Sensky T, Timberlake N, et al. Long-term efficacy of a cognitive behavioural treatment from a randomized controlled trial for patients recently diagnosed with rheumatoid arthritis. Rheumatology (Oxford) 2003;42(3):435–41.
74. Leibing E, Pfingsten M, Bartmann U, et al. Cognitive-behavioral treatment in unselected rheumatoid arthritis outpatients. Clin J Pain 1999;15(1):58–66.
75. Evers AW, Kraaimaat FW, van Riel PL, et al. Tailored cognitive-behavioral therapy in early rheumatoid arthritis for patients at risk: a randomized controlled trial. Pain 2002;100(1–2):141–53.
76. Parker JC, Smarr KL, Buckelew SP, et al. Effects of stress management on clinical outcomes in rheumatoid arthritis. Arthritis Rheum 1995;38(12):1807–18.
77. Parker J, McRae C, Smarr K, et al. Coping strategies in rheumatoid arthritis. J Rheumatol 1988;15(9):1376–83.
78. O'Leary A, Shoor S, Lorig K, et al. A cognitive-behavioral treatment for rheumatoid arthritis. Health Psychol 1988;7(6):527–44.
79. Frattaroli J. Experimental disclosure and its moderators: a meta-analysis. Psychol Bull 2006;132(6):823–65.
80. Kelley JE, Lumley MA, Leisen JC. Health effects of emotional disclosure in rheumatoid arthritis patients. Health Psychol 1997;16(4):331–40.
81. Smyth JM, Stone AA, Hurewitz A, et al. Effects of writing about stressful experiences on symptom reduction in patients with asthma or rheumatoid arthritis: a randomized trial. JAMA 1999;281(14):1304–9.

82. Wetherell MA, Byrne-Davis L, Dieppe P, et al. Effects of emotional disclosure on psychological and physiological outcomes in patients with rheumatoid arthritis: an exploratory home-based study. J Health Psychol 2005;10(2):277–85.

83. Keefe FJ, Anderson T, Lumley M, et al. A randomized, controlled trial of emotional disclosure in rheumatoid arthritis: can clinician assistance enhance the effects? Pain 2008;137(1):164–72.

84. Lan C, Lai JS, Chen SY. Tai Chi Chuan: an ancient wisdom on exercise and health promotion. Sports Med 2002;32(4):217–24.

85. Kirsteins AE, Dietz F, Hwang SM. Evaluating the safety and potential use of a weight-bearing exercise, Tai-Chi Chuan, for rheumatoid arthritis patients. Am J Phys Med Rehabil 1991;70(3):136–41.

86. Van Deusen J, Harlowe D. The efficacy of the ROM Dance Program for adults with rheumatoid arthritis. Am J Occup Ther 1987;41(2):90–5.

87. Han A, Robinson V, Judd M, et al. Tai chi for treating rheumatoid arthritis. Cochrane Database Syst Rev 2004;3:CD004849.

88. Wang C. Tai Chi improves pain and functional status in adults with rheumatoid arthritis: results of a pilot single-blinded randomized controlled trial. Med Sport Sci 2008;52:218–29.

89. Uhlig T, Fongen C, Steen E, et al. Exploring Tai Chi in rheumatoid arthritis: a quantitative and qualitative study. BMC Musculoskelet Disord 2010;11:43.

90. Uhlig T, Larsson C, Hjorth AG, et al. No improvement in a pilot study of tai chi exercise in rheumatoid arthritis. Ann Rheum Dis 2005;64(3):507–9.

91. Woolery A, Myers H, Sternlieb B, et al. A yoga intervention for young adults with elevated symptoms of depression. Altern Ther Health Med 2004;10(2): 60–3.

92. Tran MD, Holly RG, Lashbrook J, et al. Effects of Hatha Yoga practice on the health-related aspects of physical fitness. Prev Cardiol 2001;4(4):165–70.

93. Badsha H, Chhabra V, Leibman C, et al. The benefits of yoga for rheumatoid arthritis: results of a preliminary, structured 8-week program. Rheumatol Int 2009;29(12):1417–21.

94. Bosch PR, Traustadottir T, Howard P, et al. Functional and physiological effects of yoga in women with rheumatoid arthritis: a pilot study. Altern Ther Health Med 2009;15(4):24–31.

95. Haslock I, Monro R, Nagarathna R, et al. Measuring the effects of yoga in rheumatoid arthritis. Br J Rheumatol 1994;33(8):787–8.

96. Dash M, Telles S. Improvement in hand grip strength in normal volunteers and rheumatoid arthritis patients following yoga training. Indian J Physiol Pharmacol 2001;45(3):355–60.

97. Lorig KR. Arthritis self-management: a patient education program. Rehabil Nurs 1982;7(4):16–20.

98. Lorig K, Lubeck D, Kraines RG, et al. Outcomes of self-help education for patients with arthritis. Arthritis Rheum 1985;28(6):680–5.

99. Lorig KR, Mazonson PD, Holman HR. Evidence suggesting that health education for self-management in patients with chronic arthritis has sustained health benefits while reducing health care costs. Arthritis Rheum 1993;36(4): 439–46.

100. Barlow JH, Turner AP, Wright CC. A randomized controlled study of the Arthritis Self-Management Programme in the UK. Health Educ Res 2000;15(6):665–80.

101. Lindroth Y, Brattstrom M, Bellman I, et al. A problem-based education program for patients with rheumatoid arthritis: evaluation after three and twelve months. Arthritis Care Res 1997;10(5):325–32.

102. Scholten C, Brodowicz T, Graninger W, et al. Persistent functional and social benefit 5 years after a multidisciplinary arthritis training program. Arch Phys Med Rehabil 1999;80(10):1282–7.
103. Hill J, Bird H, Johnson S. Effect of patient education on adherence to drug treatment for rheumatoid arthritis: a randomised controlled trial. Ann Rheum Dis 2001;60(9):869–75.
104. Riemsma RP, Taal E, Kirwan JR, et al. Systematic review of rheumatoid arthritis patient education. Arthritis Rheum 2004;51(6):1045–59.

Epidemiology of Stress and Asthma: From Constricting Communities and Fragile Families to Epigenetics

Rosalind J. Wright, MD, MPH[a,b],*

KEYWORDS

- Epidemiology • Stress • Asthma • Epigenetics • Life course
- Transgenerational • Violence

Evidence increasingly links psychosocial stress, including early-life stress-related programming of key response systems, to asthma, atopic disorders more broadly, and lung function.[1,2] To more fully understand the potential role of psychological stress in the etiology of asthma and other allergic or inflammatory disorders, it is necessary to consider several key theoretic and methodological frameworks from social sciences, psychology, immunology, and child development and extend these to epidemiologic research. Application of recent advances in developmental biology, neurogenomics, and genomic plasticity may inform underlying mechanisms at the most fundamental level. An area of particular interest in childhood asthma research is the search for mechanisms responsible for health disparities across economic and racial/ethnic groups. The psychosocial stress model has been increasingly adopted in this regard[3] given the increasing recognition that children are being raised in social contexts that may be as detrimental to their development as established physical environmental factors associated with disease risk.[4] This review highlights the growing number of epidemiologic studies exploiting these transdisciplinary concepts

During preparation of this manuscript Dr Wright was supported by R01HL080674 and R01HL095606.

[a] Channing Laboratory, Department of Medicine, Brigham and Women's Hospital, Harvard Medical School, 181 Longwood Avenue, Boston, MA 02115, USA

[b] Department of Environmental Health, Harvard School of Public Health, 677 Huntington Avenue, Boston, MA 02115, USA

* Channing Laboratory, Department of Medicine, Brigham and Women's Hospital, Harvard Medical School, 181 Longwood Avenue, Boston, MA 02115.

E-mail address: rosalind.wright@channing.harvard.edu

to uniquely inform our understanding of the role of stress and the expression of asthma and allergy during the life course.

NEED FOR A PROSPECTIVE DEVELOPMENTAL FRAMEWORK

This overview considers the developmental origins of both asthma risk[1] and lung structure and function[2] given that both involve coordinated maturation of interrelated systems: immune, neural, and endocrine. Moreover, although the origins of chronic lung diseases are multifactorial, the underlying mechanisms leading to reduced lung function and exaggerated airway responsiveness involve chronic airway inflammation associated with a cycle of injury, repair, and remodeling.[5,6] Airway inflammation and remodeling begin and progress even in the presymptomatic state in early childhood.[7–10] Moreover, the fundamental cause of the airway inflammation is aberrant and/or excessive immune responses to various environmental factors,[5] and the most common cause of chronic airway inflammation in early childhood is arguably asthma.[11]

An important step toward identifying children at risk for costly respiratory (ie, asthma, reduced lung function) and other allergic disorders is characterizing mechanisms that lead to and maintain early predisposition. Immune and lung development occur largely in utero and during early childhood. Research continues to delineate early immunophenotypes and early airway response outcomes among children predisposed to asthma (atopic and nonatopic) and other chronic atopic disorders.[12–15] Regulatory pathways that involve the collaboration of innate and adaptive immune responses are involved. Influences of factors outside the immune system (ie, neurohormonal and autonomic nervous system (ANS) functioning) may also be involved.

Critical Periods of Development and Perinatal Programming

Plasticity is a consequence of environmental exposures in critical periods affecting key physiologic systems involved in developmental processes.[16] Although both asthma and lung function are polygenic traits,[17,18] maternal factors in particular contribute to the intergenerational correlation.[17,19,20] The risk of developing atopic disorders is particularly increased if a positive parental history of atopy is present with effects being strongest for maternal history.[19,20] Studies have also shown a greater correlation in forced expiratory volume in 1 second (FEV$_1$) and other lung function parameters between mothers (compared with fathers) and offspring.[17] In addition to heritable traits, this may be the result of perinatal programming: the influence of nongenetic or environmental factors in the perinatal period that organize or imprint physiologic systems (**Fig. 1**).[1]

Stress as a Programming Agent

The list of potential programming agents includes psychological stress. In general, stress may result in biobehavioral states (eg, posttraumatic stress disorder [PTSD], anxiety, depression) with lasting physiologic affects that influence disease risk.[21–23] Under stress, physiologic systems may operate at higher or lower levels than in normal homeostasis.[24] Disturbed regulation of maternal stress systems (eg, hypothalamus-pituitary-adrenal [HPA] axis, ANS) in pregnancy may modulate offspring immune function starting in utero.[25,26] Nonoptimal early childhood caregiving experiences may also affect these processes in children (eg, maternal psychopathology or insensitivity).[27–29]

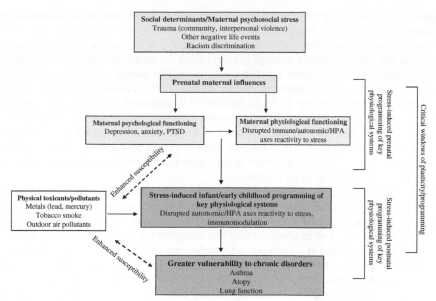

Fig. 1. Conceptual model for stress-induced perinatal programming of asthma, atopy, and lung function.

Immune Programming

Mechanisms of inflammation central to the pathophysiology of asthma phenotypes overlap and may include immune-mediated inflammation associated with a Th2-biased response[30–32] and a tendency to produce immunoglobulin E (IgE) in response to environmental stimuli (eg, allergens). The Th1-Th2 paradigm involves a complex interaction of T and B lymphocytes, resulting in the production of higher levels of particular cytokines, such as interleukin-4 (IL-4) or IL-13 and the more recently described IL-9, IL-25, and IL-31 as well as lower levels of interferon-γ [IFN-γ].[33] Evidence suggests that those with early (ie, starting in the first 2 to 3 years) sensitization to allergens are at greatest risk of developing chronic atopic disorders, airway inflammation, and obstruction (as reviewed in Ref.[2]).

However, not all asthma cases are associated with allergy and/or eosinophilic airway inflammation; neutrophilic inflammation may account for a substantial subgroup.[34,35] Thus, although this paradigm has been useful in understanding the large fraction of individuals with allergic asthma and airway inflammation, it is now accepted that the Th2-biased polarization of adaptive immunity may be only one of several axes that result in enhanced susceptibility to airway inflammation and altered reactivity.[36] Antigen-independent responses including innate immune cells (eg, bronchial epithelial cells [ECs], alveolar macrophages, and dendritic cells [DCs]) may also be important[37,38] and involve novel cytokines (eg, IL-17).[39] Factors, including stress,[1,38] that disrupt maturation of local immune networks (eg, DCs, ECs, regulatory T cells) may predispose to ongoing eosinophilic and neutrophilic inflammation. This may be manifested through the increased expression of both atopic and nonatopic persistent wheeze phenotypes in early childhood although prospective data in humans are sparse.

Immune mechanisms have their roots in utero with an immunologic bias toward a Th2 phenotype.[40–46] Immune programming can also be influenced by early postnatal environmental influences.[47,48] Consequently, researchers have begun to examine in vitro responses of peripheral blood mononuclear cells (pBMCs) to allergens or mitogens to gain a better understanding of the immunodeviations that facilitate the manifestation of asthma and atopy in response to environmental factors,[12] including stress.[49,50] Epidemiologic studies also incorporate other markers of the developing immune response (eg, IgE). Increased total IgE in cord blood, for example, has been associated with aeroallergen sensitization and the development of allergic diseases in children, particularly in those with a maternal history of atopy.[51–53] Levels of allergen-specific IgE begin to increase at age 18 to 24 months.[54] Reactivity to 2 or more allergens is detected in infants as early as 3 months with polysensitization documented after 18 to 24 months,[55] and may develop even in individuals labeled nonatopic based on a negative skin prick test (SPT).[56] The influence of stress on the timing and trajectory of these immunophenotypes and their relationship to the later development of clinical disorders has only begun to be studied.

In primates, prenatal stress affects the newborn's antigen response.[57] Evidence in prenatally stressed adult mice shows dysregulated cellular and humoral immune response on antigen challenge reflected by a Th2 adaptive response and increased IgE.[58] My group was first to prospectively link early-life caregiver stress to dysregulation of immune function in a birth cohort predisposed to allergy (ie, greater antigen-specific tumor necrosis factor [TNF]-alpha production).[49] Stress has also been associated with increased natural killer (NK) and NKT cells as well as altering their functional mechanisms,[59,60] effects correlated with changes in cortisol and ANS input.[61] Our group has also demonstrated an association between increased prenatal maternal stress and increased IL-8 and TNF-α production after microbial stimulation suggesting that stress may operate through Toll-like receptor–dependent pathways.[62]

As detailed in earlier reviews, both glucocorticoid (GC) action and sympathovagal balance play a role in immunomodulation as well as fetal and postnatal lung development.[1,2,63] Although research has advanced around the assessment of immune function in stress and asthma,[33,49,50,64] studies assessing the HPA axis[65] are scarce and none consider the autonomic response in early development (ie, pregnancy, early childhood). The HPA axis and ANS seem particularly susceptible to stress-induced programming as summarized in the next section.

HPA Axis

Maternal-fetal stress stimulates placental corticotrophin-releasing hormone (CRH), which in turn is increased in the neonatal circulation.[1,66–69] This may stimulate the fetal HPA axis, amplify GC excess and activate additional elements of the fetal stress response (ie, catecholamines) influencing developing immune function and the ANS.[26] Alterations in stress-induced maternal cortisol may influence fetal immune system development and Th2 cell predominance, perhaps through direct influence of stress hormones on cytokine production.[70,71] This may induce selective suppression of the Th1-mediated cellular immunity and trigger a shift toward Th2-mediated humoral immunity.[72] The HPA system is also influenced postnatally through child-caregiver transactions.[73] Caregiving during early development predicts the emergence of self-regulation abilities, with sensitive caregiving associated with optimal stress regulation and functioning of the child's HPA system.[1]

Studies assessing cortisol and HPA axis responses in early childhood as related to allergy and asthma risk remain sparse and none to date examine the relationship between maternal prenatal cortisol HPA axis responses (hypo- vs hyperreactivity) and childhood risk for asthma and/or allergy.[65] Bruske-Kirschbaum and colleagues[74] found an enhanced cortisol responses to stress in infants at high risk for atopic disorders based on parental history and increased level of IgE in cord blood. Ball[75] also reported a hyperreactive HPA axis in response to stress among 6-month-old infants with an allergic mother. This is in contrast to other data showing a hyporesponsive HPA axis in children who already have allergic disease.[65,76] As proposed by Bruske-Kirschbaum and colleagues,[65] it may be that the natural history in children predisposed to developing allergy and/or asthma in relation to perinatal stress have a hyperresponsive HPA axis that evolves to become hyporesponsive as time goes on and a specific disorder is expressed and becomes more chronic. Although there are inconsistencies in the literature with regard to the physiologic changes (eg, hormonal disruption) that are associated with various disease outcomes, a blunted HPA axis (more typically characterized by lower morning cortisol level, flattening of the diurnal slope) has been specifically associated with increased susceptibility to autoimmune/inflammatory diseases in overlapping research.[77,78] How disruption of the maternal prenatal HPA axis is related to childhood asthma and allergy risk and whether children of mothers with a blunted prenatal cortisol response are more likely to develop these disorders is not known. This will only be worked out through prospective epidemiologic studies incorporating biomarkers of the HPA response during these critical perinatal periods of development (for both mothers and children) and their relationship to evolving immunophenotypes and the later development of asthma and atopy.

An alternative hypothesis linking stress, neuroendocrine disruption (ie, HPA axis) and immune function considers a GC resistance model.[79,80] Insight into the cellular and molecular mechanisms underlying stress-induced steroid resistance is provided in several recent studies. Oxidative stress pathways have been implicated in the link between psychosocial stress and asthma[71] as well as steroid-resistant asthma.[81,82] This may be particularly relevant in airway inflammation where neutrophilic rather than eosinophilic inflammation predominates.[83,84] It was recently shown that oxidative stress contributes to steroid resistance in the context of neutrophilic inflammation in a mouse model of acute asthma exacerbations.[85] Psychological stress is also an oxidant and may thus operate through these same pathways.[71] Although human data in the context of lung disease are sparse in this regard, one recent cross-sectional analysis in adolescents showed that pBMCs harvested from asthmatics who perceived low parental support (ie, greater stress) were more resistant to hydrocortisone's effects on cytokine expression (IL-5, IFN-γ) and activation of eosinophils relative to asthmatics reporting higher parental support.[86] Examination of mechanisms contributing to steroid resistance in relation to perinatal stress may provide insight into the link between stress, asthma, and airway hyperresponsiveness over subsequent development.

Future studies designed to examine mechanisms underlying stress-induced programming of asthma and allergy should consider the theoretic and methodological challenges in the study of the HPA axis in early development highlighted in prior reviews.[87–91] Given the need for repeated sampling, saliva is often the preferred method given it is noninvasive and salivary cortisol follows a time course nearly identical to plasma cortisol.[92] In pregnant women, hair sampling has been proposed as a way of providing a retrospective calendar of cortisol production over the course of pregnancy.[93,94] The HPA system remains highly reactive and labile in early infancy and starts to become organized between 2 and 6 months of age through transactions between the child and caregiver.[95,96] Studies of children in naturalistic environments suggest interesting individual differences exist.[96–99] By a few months after birth, cortisol production follows a circadian rhythm and is entrained to the sleep-wake cycle.[100] However, individuals may vary in the age at which they acquire particular components of this variation (eg, diurnal rhythm, cortisol-awakening response).[95,101] It has been proposed that the age of appearance (ie, early vs late), stability, and curve profile may be characteristic of developmentally distinct groups of infants and may have differential influence on subsequent health.[95,102] Children's sleep-wake cycle varies greatly over the day in early development and, as in older samples, analyses must consider time from awakening but also napping characteristics (eg, time of napping, total number, and duration of naps).[103] There are also gender effects.[104] Moreover, different methods of analysis may contribute to different conclusions related to profiles throughout the day and age of appearance of the circadian rhythm.[95,105] Understanding this complexity and accounting for these factors in research examining alterations in adaptations of HPA axis activity in relation to perinatal stress and subsequent disease risk (eg, asthma) is important; not doing so may obscure true patterns and associations.

When incorporating salivary collection protocols into larger epidemiologic studies,[90,91] the burden on participants and staff in light of other activities, and balancing the number of samples needed to accurately assess the HPA response versus the likelihood that the most interesting participants (eg, those most stressed, mothers/children with psychopathology) may be overwhelmed, must be considered. How samples are collected may need to vary with the age and developmental stage of the participant (eg, absorbent cotton rolls, passive drool, and so forth), each with their own tradeoffs. Possible confounders, mediators, and moderators of stress effects relevant to the life stage being examined also need to be addressed. For example, dysregulation of the HPA axis in pregnant women (and older children) may differ based on current psychological functioning (depression, PTSD) as different biologic profiles may be associated with specific psychopathology.[106,107] Also in pregnant women, stage of gestation (weeks pregnant at time of cortisol sampling) and other prenatal factors (eg, prenatal alcohol and tobacco use, maternal body mass index calculated as weight in kilograms divided by the square of height in meters) may be important (for reviews see Refs.[108,109]). Child temperament,[110] an individual characteristic that dictates the tendency to express particular emotions with a certain intensity, is an important factor to consider in early child development.

Autonomic Reactivity

Animal and human studies support the connection between an adverse intrauterine environment as well as experiences in early postnatal life and alterations of ANS functioning (eg, sympathovagal balance).[111–114] The ANS, in turn, plays an important role in immunoregulation.[115–117] Animal research suggests that neural control of airway smooth muscle and irritant receptor systems are sensitive to environmental programming.[111] Respiratory and vagal systems undergo postnatal maturation to establish an integration of respiratory and cardiovascular function.[118,119] Much remains to be learned about the vulnerability of these systems to perinatal environmental influences and early programming.[120] In humans, autonomic responses show developmental changes with relative stability between 6 and 12 months of age.[121] It seems plausible that disruption of neuroendocrine and vagal antiinflammatory pathways may predispose some individuals to immunodeviations and consequent excessive inflammatory responses that may result in altered respiratory responses in early life. The balance between functional parasympathetic and sympathetic activity in relation to emotional stimuli and immune function may be important for airway inflammation and enhanced airway reactivity to a psychological stressor, although this has not been examined in human research. My group has demonstrated differential stress reactivity as indexed by prenatal HPA axis disruption[122] and cardiorespiratory parameters in infancy[123] in an urban pregnancy cohort designed to study the effects of prenatal maternal and early-life stress on urban childhood asthma risk. Future analyses will examine links between stress-elicited changes in these systems and asthma risk and lung function as these children get older.

Prenatal stress increases allergen-induced airway inflammation in mice offspring.[124,125] Similarly, allergen aerosol challenge is associated with increased airway hyperresponsiveness in prenatally stressed mice.[58] Others show exacerbations in airway inflammation in ovalbumin-sensitized rats after repeated psychosocial challenge.[126–130] In humans, reversible airway obstruction has been demonstrated during psychological challenge; cholinergic blockade supports a vagal origin.[131,132] Negative affect in particular increase airway resistance.[133] Vagal excitation to the airways is the supported mechanism.[134] Airway responses to induction of depressed mood is correlated with increased respiratory sinus arrhythmia in asthmatics.[135,136] Individuals with a tendency toward greater vagal system response to distress may be prone to exaggerated airway narrowing in such situations, although this has not been studied in young children.

Need for the Integration of Stress Systems in Research

These data suggest that stress-elicited disruption of interrelated systems (autonomic, neuroendocrine, and immune systems) may lead to increased vulnerability to early allergic sensitization, which predisposes to persistent atopic disorders. To date, most studies examining links between stress-elicited disruption of physiologic systems and various health outcomes have examined one system in isolation from the others. However, recent findings specifically related to HPA and ANS functioning highlight the need to consider these systems simultaneously because of interactive influences.[137–139] Studies that do not assess the interactions among these systems may obscure stress-related influences on asthma and allergy expression.

GENETICS

Most advances in our knowledge of the genetic and molecular events underlying the neurobiology of the stress response have occurred in animal models[140] and psychiatric outcomes in humans.[141] These animal data suggest that studies to determine the role of genetics in modifying the risk of the social/physical environment experienced through psychological stress may further inform pathways through which stress may affect asthma expression. Genetic factors of potential importance include those that influence immune development and airway inflammation in early life, corticosteroid regulatory genes, adrenergic system regulatory genes, biotransformation genes, and cytokine pathway genes.

Genes expressed in the lung involved in determining the effects of oxidative stress, specifically the glutathione S-transferase, have been found to be functionally and clinically significant in recent studies in relation to atopic risk. Gilliland and colleagues[142] found that specific GSTP1 variants are associated with increased histamine and IgE responses to air pollution oxidants and allergens in vivo. Maternal genetics related to oxidative stress genes may influence the child's atopic risk beginning in utero[143] Variants of the GC receptor gene may contribute to interindividual variability in HPA axis activity and GC sensitivity in response to stress.[144,145] Studies related to factors regulating the feedback mechanisms involved in the GC response to stress are also of interest.[146] A recent study examined polymorphisms of the TNF-alpha promoter region (TNF-308G/A) and linked specific variants to increased C-reactive protein (CRP), a proinflammatory marker.[147] These are potentially interesting candidate genes to include in future studies of risk for atopic disease. Such studies that consider gene × environment interactions (ie, stress by pathway genes) may inform specific mechanisms related to stress and atopy.

EPIGENETICS: A FUNDAMENTAL PROGRAMMING MECHANISM

Programming effects of stress on respiratory outcomes may operate at a more funda-mental molecular level, through epigenetic programming. Epigenetics may be at the roots of developmental plasticity imprinting environmental experiences on the fixed genome,[148] although data are scare for respiratory health and allergic disorders.[149,150] Determining the range of environmental exposures that affect the epigenome during development was a research priority identified at the recent National Heart Lung and Blood Institute *Pediatric Pulmonary Disease Strategic Planning Workshop*.[151] DNA methylation is an adaptable epigenetic mechanism that modifies genome func-tion by the addition of methyl groups to cytosine to form 5-methyl-cytosine. DNA methylation marks are largely established early in life[16] and may ensure stable regula-tion that mediates persistent changes in biologic and behavioral phenotypes over the lifespan. DNA methylation of many genes changes with disease status and in response to environmental signals including chemical exposures such as diet, drugs, and toxins. Recent findings also implicate psychological stress as shown in behavioral studies that demonstrated epigenetic changes during fear conditioning[152,153] and from evidence of epigenetic programming related to maternal care.[154,155]

The epigenome may be particularly sensitive to dysregulation in early development when DNA synthesis rates are highest. Genes involved in HPA axis functioning seem particularly susceptible to stress-related programming.[73] These include GC receptor expression, the activation of which alters HPA activity through negative feedback inhi-bition. The human GC receptor promoter region is extensively methylated with diverse methylation profiles demonstrated in normal donors.[156] The intracellular access of GCs to their receptors is also modulated by the 11β-hydroxysteroid dehydrogenase (11βHSD) enzymes, which interconvert biologically active 11β-hydroxyglucocorticoids and inactive 11-ketosteroids.[157] Although compromised 11βHSD2 activity can be caused by loss of function mutations of the gene encoding 11βHSD2, the frequency of such mutations is extremely low. Thus, other mechanisms accounting for the inter-individual variability in 11βHSD2 enzyme activity should be considered. The 11βHSD2 promoter comprises a highly (G + C)-rich (or GC-rich) core, contains more than 80% GC, lacks a TATA-like element, and has 2 typical CpG islands raising the possibility that methylation may play a role in the epigenetically determined interindividual variable expression of 11βHSD2. Another candidate pathway implicated in both airway inflam-mation[158] and autonomic response[159] is the nitric oxide (NO) signaling pathways. Alter-ations of NO expression occur in the context of psychological stress and stress-related behaviors.[160] The inducible nitric oxide synthase (NOS) genes are also susceptible to epigenetic programming.[161]

The notion that variability in methylation between individuals may reflect an impor-tant epigenetic mechanism is suggested by recent studies in both animals and humans. Epigenetic modulation of the 11βHSD2 gene has been demonstrated recently in a rodent model and cultured cell lines,[162] although epigenetic regulation of this gene is not well characterized in humans. Weaver and colleagues[163] have demonstrated differential methylation patterns of the Ngfi-A-binding site in GC receptor promoter 1_7 in the rat brain in offspring that had received poor maternal care versus those that had received better maternal care. When pups were cross-fostered between dams providing good or poor postnatal care, the pups developed the epigenome of the foster mother. This same group reported increased methylation in a neuron-specific GC receptor (NR3C1) promoter as well as decreased levels of GC receptor mRNA from hippocampus tissue obtained from suicide victims with a history of childhood abuse.[164] Recent human data demonstrate that methylation of exon 1F in fetal cord blood was sensitive to maternal mood in the perinatal period and the infant's HPA stress reactivity.[165]

In summary, genetic and epigenetic studies tell us that exposure to altered GC receptor response through early development, even beginning in utero, programs major changes in the endogenous neuroendocrine and immune mechanisms that may, in turn, lead to increased vulnerability to asthma. Whether alterations in DNA methylation underlie stress-induced phenotypic plasticity related to lung structure and function or asthma risk remains largely unexplored. It will be important to begin to understand factors related to developmental programming of GC sensitivity during critical periods of development that may play a role in disease etiology as well as subsequent morbidity.

Characterizing Stress in Epidemiologic Studies

The cause of health problems is increasingly recognized as a result of the complex interplay of influences operating at several levels, including the individual, the family, and the community (**Fig. 2**). Ecological views on health recognize that individual-level health risks and behaviors have multilevel determinants, in part influenced by the social context within which people live.[166] That is, chronic stress experiences are significantly influenced by the characteristics of the families, homes, and communities in which we live.[167,168] Both physical and social factors can be a source of environmental demands that contribute to stress experienced by populations living in a particular area.[169]

Taking a multilevel approach to examining stress effects on asthma expression may be particularly relevant to the understanding of disparities based on race/ethnicity and socioeconomic status.[168] This includes an environmental justice perspective underscoring the role of structural and macrosocial forces that shape exposure and vulnerability to diseases may better inform the complex social patterning of asthma.[168] According to this framework, asthma rates are higher and the associated morbidity is greater among the poor because they bear a disproportionate burden of exposure to suboptimal, unhealthy environmental conditions. Upstream social and economic factors determine differential exposures to relevant asthma pathogens and

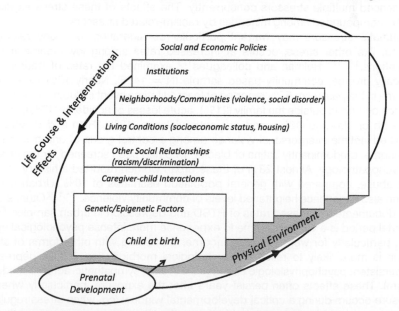

Fig. 2. Characterizing stress across the life course: an ecological approach.

toxicants.[170] Also, understanding the upstream factors (eg, social and economic policies) that contribute to the varying social conditions for populations and individuals being studied will better inform needed interventions.

Thus, a challenge in any epidemiologic study linking stress to health is how to measure and characterize the stressor(s). An important consideration is the prevalence of the stressor(s) of interest in a particular population. The decision can also be theoretically guided by our empirical understanding of how certain stressor characteristics influence behavioral and physiologic correlates that may have a particular pathogenic effect. The latter may vary based on the condition being considered and our understanding of the natural history of the disorder being considered. Although it can be acknowledged that there are inconsistencies in the literature with regard to the physiologic changes (eg, hormonal disruption) that are associated with various disease outcomes, a blunted HPA axis (more typically characterized by lower morning cortisol level and flattening of the diurnal slope) has been specifically associated with increased susceptibility to autoimmune/inflammatory diseases.[77,78] This is also a pattern frequently described in the setting of extreme chronic stress that includes traumatic stressors (even occurring remote to the timing of study) and cumulative stressors that are chronic or co-occur. Stress exposure can be conceptualized as extreme if the individual experiences (1) multiple stressors in the same period, (2) chronic stressors in repeated developmental periods, or (3) the nature of the stress is extreme (eg, trauma).

Given the earlier discussion on perinatal programming, experiences of women of child-bearing age is particularly relevant. Women with low income, especially ethnic minorities, report greater and more frequent exposure to chronic extreme stress and greater psychological distress as a result. For example, in a study examining stressors immediately before or during pregnancy among a sample of 143,452 women,[171] stress exposure increased as income decreased, with 57% of women on low income experiencing at least 1 chronic stressor (eg, economic hardship 37%, job loss 19%, separation or divorce 15%, incarceration of partner 8%, and domestic violence 5%); 29% experienced multiple stressors concurrently. The effects of these stress exposures may be compounded among minorities by racism-related stressors.

Traumatic stressors may warrant particular consideration for many reasons.[73] Trauma, like other stress, occurs at increased rates among low-income minority populations.[172,173] Holman and colleagues[173] examined the rates of trauma in an ethnically diverse, community-based sample (N = 1456). Nearly 10% experienced a trauma in the past year; 57% reported at least 1 lifetime event including interpersonal violence occurring outside the family (21%), acute losses or accidents (17%), witnessing death or violence (13%), and domestic violence (12%). Hien and Bukszpan[174] examined lifetime interpersonal violence among a control group of urban women on low income, predominantly Latina or blacks, who had been screened for the absence of psychopathology. Almost 28% of these urban women reported a history of childhood abuse, compared with general population estimates of 10%. Urban minority women also experience heightened levels of community violence.[175,176] Other studies have documented increased rates of PTSD and depression in urban samples.[73] The perinatal period is a vulnerable time to experience more intense psychological symptoms, particularly for women on low income. Compared with other forms of stress, trauma is more likely to result in psychological morbidity (eg, PTSD, depression) and persistent psychophysiologic changes (HPA axis, sympathetic-adrenal-medullary system). These effects often persist years after the exposure, particularly when the exposure occurs during a critical developmental window (eg, when stress regulatory systems are becoming consolidated in the mother).

Life Course Perspective and Intergenerational Effects

Other studies provide evidence supporting the intergenerational transmission of psycho-physiologic vulnerability in traumatized populations. Although studies of maternal stress and infant outcomes typically examine events occurring during pregnancy, we recently considered stress (interpersonal trauma [IPT]) during the mother's life course in relation to early immune markers in their children.[177] The life-course perspective posits that some stressors may influence health through 2 mechanisms, early programming and cumulative pathways, in addition to more immediate effects. Early programming may occur if exposures during sensitive developmental periods in the mother have lasting psychobiologic sequelae. Exposure to IPT in earlier life can generate disrupted physiologic stress responses even several years after the trauma. Thus, maternal IPT may be linked to infant health through more latent effects (ie, lasting effects from abuse in childhood/adolescence), proximate effects (ie, trauma experienced in or around the pregnancy) and cumulative life-course effects (ie, allostatic load of accumulated traumas in the mother's life). We investigated the relationship between maternal IPT experienced in her life course and total IgE in cord blood, a biomarker of atopic risk at birth, in an urban population-based study. We demonstrated that infants born to mothers with chronic trauma exposure (ie, both early in life and more proximate to the pregnancy) would be at greatest risk of expressing increased IgE.

Constricting Communities

Indicators of neighborhood disadvantage, characterized by the presence of several area-level stressors including poverty, unemployment/underemployment, percentage of unskilled laborers, limited social capital or social cohesion, substandard housing, and high crime/violence exposure rates, have been investigated in relation to urban children's development.[168] Such stress is chronic and can affect all individuals in a given environment regardless of their individual-level risks.

For example, accumulating evidence suggests that community violence may contribute to the burden of asthma in urban populations.[5] Increased exposure is associated with more symptom days,[10] higher hospitalization rates,[11] increased asthma prevalence among children in communities with both increased levels of crime/violence and other environmental hazards (ie, ambient air pollutants),[12] and increased risk of wheezing at ages 2 to 3 years.[13] In a longitudinal multilevel study including 2071 children aged 0 to 9 years at enrollment from the Project on Human Development in Chicago Neighborhoods (PHDCN), we demonstrated a significant association between exposure to community violence and increased risk for asthma development in urban children.[178] This association was robust in controlling for important individual-level factors (race/ethnicity, socioeconomic status, maternal health behaviors, family violence), and neighborhood-level confounders (concentrated disadvantage, social disorder, and collective efficacy).

Housing Stressors

Recent reviews highlight several subjective housing characteristics that have been linked to adverse psychological outcomes. This subjective emotional dimension of housing may influence asthma outcomes,[179] although this is only starting to be empirically explored.[180]

Family Factors

There have been several examples from the asthma epidemiology literature showing associations between early caregiver stress and the development of asthmatic phenotypes in early childhood.[181,182] We recently demonstrated that maternal ability to maintain positive caregiving processes in the context of even more extreme stress may buffer the effects on child asthma risk. We examined the prospective relationship between maternal intimate partner violence (IPV) and asthma onset in children in the Fragile Families and Child Wellbeing Study (N = 3117), a birth cohort. Maternal reports of IPV were assessed after the child's birth and at 12 and 36 months. Mothers also indicated how many days a week they participated in activities with the child and the amount and type of educational/recreational toys available for the child. Maternal reports of physician-diagnosed asthma by age 36 months was the outcome. In adjusted analysis, children of mothers experiencing IPV chronically (at all time periods), compared with those not exposed, had a 2-fold increased risk of developing asthma. In stratified analysis, children of mothers experiencing IPV and low levels of mother-child activities (relative risk [RR] 2.7, 95% confidence interval [CI] 1.6, 4.7) had a significant increased risk for asthma. Those exposed to IPV and high levels of mother-child activities had a lower risk for asthma (RR 1.6, 95% CI 0.9, 3.2). Earlier the relationship between parental support and GC resistance in adolescent asthmatics was discussed.[86]

Although beyond the scope of the current discussion given space limitations, the developmental timing of exposures during the life course relative to specific asthma outcomes must be considered whether individual or contextual factors are being considered. Factors leading to the onset, remission, or persistence of asthma during the life course may be influenced by social experiences and physical exposures beginning in utero, a series of social and biologic experiences initiated by early childhood exposure, or cumulative exposure to toxic biologic or social factors at critical periods of development (see **Fig. 2**). It is important to consider stress at these multiple levels given that they are interrelated throughout the life course. If we can understand at what level stress is occurring and perhaps has the greatest effect on asthma expression, this may inform the most effective interventions.

Stress-enhancing Effects on Physical Environmental Exposures

Because of the covariance in exposures and evidence that social stress and other environmental toxins (eg, pollutants, tobacco smoke) may influence common physiologic pathways (eg, oxidative stress, proinflammatory immune pathways, autonomic disruption), understanding the potential synergistic effects promises to more completely inform children's asthma risk.[4] Epidemiologic studies have demonstrated synergistic effects of stress and air pollution on asthma expression among children and adolescents.[183–185] We need to better understand how the physical and psychological demands of living in a relatively deprived environment may potentiate an individual's susceptibility to cumulative exposures across these domains.

SUMMARY

The evidence points toward the need to consider social environmental factors (ie, stress) as mainstream in asthma epidemiologic research. The likelihood of multiple mechanistic pathways with complex interdependencies must be considered when examining the integrative influence of stress independently, as well as the interaction of social and physical environmental toxins on asthma and atopy. Because these factors tend to cluster in the most socially disadvantaged, this line of research may better inform the etiology of growing health disparities. Design of future epidemiologic studies and effective intervention programs will need to address social stress and physical environmental toxins jointly to affect outcomes on a public health scale more effectively.

REFERENCES

1. Wright RJ. Prenatal maternal stress and early caregiving experiences: implications for childhood asthma risk. Paediatr Perinat Epidemiol 2007;21:8–14.
2. Wright RJ. Perinatal stress and early life programming of lung structure and function. Biol Psychol 2010;84:46–56.
3. Gee GC, Payne-Sturges DC. Environmental health disparities: a framework integrating psychosocial and environmental concepts. Environ Health Perspect 2004;112:1645–53.
4. Wright RJ. Moving towards making social toxins mainstream in children's environmental health. Curr Opin Pediatr 2009;21:222–9.
5. Holt PG, Upham JW, Sly PD. Contemporaneous maturation of immunologic and respiratory functions during early childhood: implications for development of asthma prevention strategies. J Allergy Clin Immunol 2005;116:16–24 [quiz: 25].
6. Holgate ST. Asthma: a dynamic disease of inflammation and repair. In: Chadwick DJ, Cardew G, editors. The rising trends in asthma. Chichester (UK): John Wiley; 1997. p. 5–34.
7. Pohunek P, Warner JO, Turzikova J, et al. Markers of eosinophilic inflammation and tissue re-modelling in children before clinically diagnosed bronchial asthma. Pediatr Allergy Immunol 2005;16:43–51.
8. van den Toorn LM, Overbeek SE, de Jongste JC, et al. Airway inflammation is present during clinical remission of atopic asthma. Am J Respir Crit Care Med 2001;164:2107–13.
9. Morgan WJ, Stern DA, Sherrill DL, et al. Outcome of asthma and wheezing in the first 6 years of life: follow-up through adolescence. Am J Respir Crit Care Med 2005;172:1253–8.
10. Rasmussen F, Taylor DR, Flannery EM, et al. Risk factors for airway remodeling in asthma manifested by a low postbronchodilator FEV1/vital capacity ratio: a longitudinal population study from childhood to adulthood. Am J Respir Crit Care Med 2002;165:1480–8.
11. Prescott SL. The development of respiratory inflammation in children. Paediatr Respir Rev 2006;7:89–96.
12. Heaton T, Rowe J, Turner S, et al. An immunoepidemiological approach to asthma: identification of in-vitro T-cell response patterns associated with different wheezing phenotypes in children. Lancet 2005;365:142–9.
13. Saglani S, Bush A. The early-life origins of asthma. Curr Opin Allergy Clin Immunol 2007;7:83–90.
14. Williams HE, Flohr C. How epidemiology has challenged 3 prevailing concepts about atopic dermatitis. J Allergy Clin Immunol 2006;118:209–13.
15. Hahn EL, Bacharier LB. The atopic march: the pattern of allergic disease development in childhood. Immunol Allergy Clin North Am 2005;25:231–46.
16. Feinberg AP. Phenotypic plasticity and the epigenetics of human disease. Nature 2007;447:433–40.
17. Holberg CJ, Morgan WJ, Wright AL, et al. Differences in familial segregation of FEV1 between asthmatic and nonasthmatic families: role of maternal component. Am J Respir Crit Care Med 1998;158:162–9.
18. Kumar A, Ghosh B. Genetics of asthma: a molecular biologist perspective. Clin Mol Allergy 2009;7:7.
19. Litonjua AA, Carey VJ, Burge HA, et al. Parental history and the risk for childhood asthma. Does mother confer more risk than father? Am J Respir Crit Care Med 1998;158:176–81.

20. Bjerg A, Hedman L, Perzanowski MS, et al. Family history of asthma and atopy: in-depth analyses of the impact on asthma and wheeze in 7- to 8-year-old children. Pediatrics 2007;120:741–8.
21. Cohen S, Herbert T. Health psychology: psychological factors and physical disease from the perspective of human psychoneuroimmunology. Annu Rev Psychol 1996;47:113–42.
22. Cohen S, Janicki-Deverts D, Miller GE. Psychological stress and disease. JAMA 2007;298:1685–7.
23. Cacioppo JT, Berntson CG, Malarkey WB, et al. Autonomic, neuroendocrine, and immune responses to psychological stress: the reactivity hypothesis. Ann N Y Acad Sci 1998;840:664–73.
24. McEwen BS. Protective and damaging effects of stress mediators: the good and bad sides of the response to stress. Metabolism 2002;51:2–4.
25. de Weerth C, Buitelaar JK. Physiological stress reactivity in human pregnancy – a review. Neurosci Biobehav Rev 2005;29:295–312.
26. Arck PC, Knackstedt MK, Blois SM. Current insights and future perspectives on neuro-endocrine-immune circuitry challenging pregnancy maintenance and fetal health. J Reproductionsmed Endokrinol 2006;3:98–102.
27. Vallee M, Mayo W, Dellu F, et al. Prenatal stress induces high anxiety and post-natal handling induces low anxiety in adult offspring: correlation with stress-induced corticosterone secretion. J Neurosci 1997;17:2626–36.
28. Liu D, Diorio J, Tannenbaum B, et al. Maternal care, hippocampal gluccocorticoid receptors, and hypothalamic-pituitary-adrenal response to stress. Science 1997;277:1659–62.
29. Anisman H, Zaharia MD, Meaney MJ, et al. Do early-life events permanently alter behavioral and hormonal responses to stressors? Int J Dev Neurosci 1998;16:149–64.
30. Mossman TR, Coffman RL. TH1 and TH2 cells: different patterns of lymphokine secretion lead to different functional properties. Annu Rev Immunol 1989;7: 145–73.
31. Mossman TR, Sad S. The expanding universe of T-cell subsets: Th1, Th2 and more. Immunol Today 1996;17:138–46.
32. Robinson DS, Hamid Q, Ying S, et al. Predominant Th2 like bronchoalveolar T-lymphocyte population in atopic asthma. N Engl J Med 1992;326:298–304.
33. Commins SP, Borish L, Steinke JW. Immunologic messenger molecules: cytokines, interferons, and chemokines. J Allergy Clin Immunol 2010;125:S53–72.
34. Fahy JV. Eosinophilic and neutrophilic inflammation in asthma: insights from clinical studies. Proc Am Thorac Soc 2009;6:256–9.
35. Haldar P, Pavord ID. Noneosinophilic asthma: a distinct clinical and pathologic phenotype. J Allergy Clin Immunol 2007;119:1043–52.
36. Woodruff PG, Modrek B, Choy DF, et al. Th2-driven inflammation defines major sub-phenotypes of asthma. Am J Respir Crit Care Med 2009;180(5): 994–50.
37. Suarez CJ, Parker NJ, Finn PW. Innate immune mechanism in allergic asthma. Curr Allergy Asthma Rep 2008;8:451–9.
38. Joachim RA, Handjiski B, Blois SM, et al. Stress-induced neurogenic inflammation in murine skin skews dendritic cells towards maturation and migration. Key role of intercellular adhesion molecule-1/leukocyte function-associated antigen interactions. Am J Pathol 2008;173:1379–88.
39. Cua DJ, Tato CM. Innate IL-17-producing cells: the sentinels of the immune system. Nat Rev Immunol 2010;10(7):479–89.

40. Peden DB. Development of atopy and asthma: candidate environmental influences and important periods of exposure. Environ Health Perspect 2000;108:475–82.
41. Devereux G, Barker RN, Seaton A. Antenatal determinants of neonatal immune responses to allergens. Clin Exp Allergy 2002;32:43–50.
42. Devereux G, Seaton A, Barker RN. In utero priming of allergen-specific helper T cells. Clin Exp Allergy 2001;31:1686–95.
43. Prescott SL, Macaubas C, Holt BJ, et al. Transplacental priming of the human immune system to environmental allergens: universal skewing of initial T cell responses toward the Th2 cytokine profile. J Immunol 1998;160:4730–7.
44. Miles EA, Warner JA, Jones AC, et al. Peripheral blood mononuclear cell proliferative responses in the first year of life in babies born to allergic parents. Clin Exp Allergy 1996;26:780–8.
45. Liao SY, Liao TN, Chiang BL, et al. Decreased production of IFN gamma and increased production of IL-6 by cord blood mononuclear cells of newborns with a high risk of allergy. Clin Exp Allergy 1996;26:397–405.
46. Tang ML, Kemp AS, Thorburn J, et al. Reduced interferon-gamma secretion in neonates and subsequent atopy. Lancet 1994;344:983–5.
47. Taussig LM, Wright AL, Holberg CJ, et al. Tucson children's respiratory study: 1980 to present. J Allergy Clin Immunol 2003;111:661–75.
48. Willwerth BM, Schaub B, Tantisira KG, et al. Prenatal, perinatal, and heritable influences on cord blood immune responses. Ann Allergy Asthma Immunol 2006;96:445–53.
49. Wright RJ, Finn PW, Contreras JP, et al. Chronic caregiver stress and IgE expression, allergen-induced proliferation and cytokine profiles in a birth cohort predisposed to atopy. J Allergy Clin Immunol 2004;113:1051–7.
50. Chen E, Fisher EB, Bacharier LB, et al. Socioeconomic status, stress, and immune markers in adolescents with asthma. Psychosom Med 2003;65: 984–92.
51. Tariq SM, Arshad SH, Matthews SM, et al. Elevated cord serum IgE increases the risk of aeroallergen sensitization without increasing respiratory allergic symptoms in early childhood. Clin Exp Allergy 1999;29:1042–8.
52. Odelram H, Bjorksten B, Leander E, et al. Predictors of atopy in newborn babies. Allergy 1995;50:585–92.
53. Halken S. Early sensitization and development of allergic airway disease – risk factors and predictors. Paediatr Respir Rev 2003;4:128–34.
54. Rowntree S, Cogswell JJ, Platts-Mills TA, et al. Development of IgE and IgG antibodies to food and inhalant allergens in children at risk of allergic disease. Arch Dis Child 1985;60:727–35.
55. Johnke H, Norberg LA, Vach W, et al. Patterns of sensitization in infants and its relation to atopic dermatitis. Pediatr Allergy Immunol 2006;17:591–600.
56. Burney PG, Newson RB, Burrows MS, et al. The effects of allergens in outdoor air on both atopic and nonatopic subjects with airway disease. Allergy 2008;63:542–6.
57. Coe CL, Lubach GR, Karaszewski JW. Prenatal stress and immune recognition of self and nonself in the primate neonate. Biol Neonate 1999;76:301–10.
58. Pincus-Knackstedt MK, Joachim RA, Blois SM, et al. Prenatal stress enhances susceptibility of murine adult offspring toward airway inflammation. J Immunol 2006;177:8484–92.
59. Lutgendorf SK, Moore MB, Bradley S, et al. Distress and expression of natural killer receptors on lymphocytes. Brain Behav Immun 2005;19:185–94.
60. Oya H, Kawamura T, Shimizu T, et al. The differential effect of stress on natural killer T (NKT) and NK cell function. Clin Exp Immunol 2000;121:384–90.

61. Sagiyama K, Tsuchida M, Kawamura H, et al. Age-related bias in function of natural killer T cells and granulocytes after stress: reciprocal association of steroid hormones and sympathetic nerves. Clin Exp Immunol 2004;135:56–63.

62. Wright RJ, Visness CM, Calatroni A, et al. Prenatal maternal stress and cord blood innate and adaptive cytokine responses in an inner-city population. Am J Respir Crit Care Med 2010;182(1):25–33.

63. Bolt RJ, van Weissenbruch MM, Lafever HN, et al. Glucocorticoids and lung development in the fetus and preterm infant. Pediatr Pulmonol 2001;32:76–91.

64. Chen E, Miller GE. Stress and inflammation in exacerbations of asthma. Brain Behav Immun 2007;21:993–9.

65. Buske-Kirschbaum A. Cortisol responses to stress in allergic children: interaction with the immune response. Neuroimmunomodulation 2009;16:325–32.

66. Seckl J. Glucocorticoids, feto-placental 11-beta-hydroxysteroid dehydrogenase type 2, and the early life origins of adult disease. Steroids 1997;62:89–94.

67. Seckl JR. Glucocorticoid programming of the fetus: adult phenotypes and molecular mechanisms. Mol Cell Endocrinol 2001;185:61–71.

68. Reinisch JM, Simon NG, Karwo WG, et al. Prenatal exposure to prednisone in humans and animals retards intra-uterine growth. Science 1978;202.

69. Goland RS, Jozak S, Warren WB, et al. Elevated levels of umbilical cord plasma corticotropin-releasing hormone in growth-related fetuses. J Clin Endocrinol Metab 1993;77:1174–9.

70. von Hertzen LC. Maternal stress and T-cell differentiation of the developing immune system: possible implications for the development of asthma and atopy. J Allergy Clin Immunol 2002;109:923–8.

71. Wright RJ. Stress and atopic disorders. J Allergy Clin Immunol 2005;116: 1301–6.

72. Elenkov IJ, Iezzoni DG, Daly A, et al. Cytokine dysregulation, inflammation and well-being. Neuroimmunomodulation 2005;12:255–69.

73. Wright R, Bosquet EM. Maternal stress and perinatal programming in the expression of atopy. Expert Rev Clin Immunol 2008;4:535–8.

74. Buske-Kirschbaum A, Fischbach S, Rauh W, et al. Increased responsiveness of the hypothalamus-pituitary-adrenal (HPA) axis to stress in newborns with atopic disposition. Psychoneuroendocrinology 2004;29:705–11.

75. Ball TM. Cortisol circadian rhythms and stress responses in infants at risk of allergic disease. Neuroimmunomodulation 2006;13:294–300.

76. Landstra AM, Postma DS, Boezen M, et al. Role of serum cortisol levels in children with asthma. Am J Respir Crit Care Med 2002;165:708–12.

77. Eskandari F, Webster JI, Sternberg EM. Neural immune pathways and their connection to inflammatory diseases. Arthritis Res Ther 2003;5:251–65.

78. Raison CL, Miller AH. When not enough is too much: the role of insufficient glucocorticoid signaling in the pathophysiology of stress-related disorders. Am J Psychiatry 2003;260:1554–65.

79. Miller GE, Cohen S, Ritchey AK. Chronic psychological stress and the regulation of pro-inflammatory cytokines: a glucocorticoid-resistance model. Health Psychol 2002;21:531–41.

80. Haczku A, Panettieri RA. Social stress and asthma: the role of corticosteroid insensitivity. J Allergy Clin Immunol 2010;125:550–8.

81. Marwick JA, Wallis G, Meja K, et al. Oxidative stress modulates theophylline effects on steroid responsiveness. Biochem Biophys Res Commun 2008;377:797–802.

82. Adcock IM, Barnes PJ. Molecular mechanisms of corticosteroid resistance. Chest 2008;134:394–401.

83. Wenzel SE, Schwartz LB, Langmack EL, et al. Evidence that severe asthma can be divided pathologically into two inflammatory subtypes with distinct physiologic and clinical characteristics. Am J Respir Crit Care Med 1999;160:1001–8.

84. Bush A. How early do airway inflammation and remodeling occur? Allergol Int 2008;57:11–9.

85. Ito K, Herbert C, Diegle JS, et al. Steroid-resistant neutrophilic inflammation in a mouse model of an acute exacerbation of asthma. Am J Respir Cell Mol Biol 2008;39:543–50.

86. Miller GE, Gaudin A, Zysk E, et al. Parental support and cytokine activity in childhood asthma: the role of glucocorticoid sensitivity. J Allergy Clin Immunol 2009; 123:824–30.

87. Field T, Diego M. Cortisol: the culprit prenatal stress variable. Int J Neurosci 2008;118:1181–205.

88. Levine A, Zagoory-Sharon O, Feldman R, et al. Measuring cortisol in human psychobiological studies. Physiol Behav 2007;90:43–53.

89. Egliston KA, McMahan C, Austin MP. Stress in pregnancy and infant HPA axis function: conceptual and methodological issues relating to the use of salivary cortisol as an outcome measure. Psychoneuroendocrinology 2007;32:1–13.

90. Adam EK, Kumari M. Assessing salivary cortisol in large-scale, epidemiological research. Psychoneuroendocrinology 2009;34:1423–36.

91. Adam EK, Doane LD, Mendelsohn K. Spit, sweat, and tears: measuring biological data in naturalistic settings. In: Hargittai E, editor. Research confidential: solutions to problems most social scientists pretend they never have. Ann Arbor (MI): University of Michigan Press; 2009. p. 3–37.

92. Dom LD, Lucke JF, Loucks TL, et al. Salivary cortisol reflects serum cortisol: analysis of circadian profiles. Ann Clin Biochem 2007;44:281–4.

93. Kirschbaum C, Tietze A, Skoluda N, et al. Hair as a retrospective calendar of cortisol production – increased cortisol incorporation into hair in the third trimester of pregnancy. Psychoneuroendocrinology 2009;34(1):32–7.

94. Kalra S, Einarson A, Karaskov T, et al. The relationship between stress and hair cortisol in healthy pregnant women. Clin Invest Med 2007;30:E103–7.

95. de Weerth C, Zijl RH, Buitelaar JK. Development of cortisol circadian rhythm in infancy. Early Hum Dev 2003;73:39–52.

96. Gunnar MR, Quevedo K. The neurobiology of stress and development. Annu Rev Psychol 2007;58:145–73.

97. Flinn MV. Evolution an ontogeny of stress response to social challenge in the human child. Dev Rev 2006;26:138–74.

98. Lupien SJ, King S, Meaney MJ, et al. Child's stress hormone levels correlate with mother's socioeconomic status and depressive state. Biol Psychiatry 2000;48:976–80.

99. Suglia SF, Staudenmayer J, Cohen S, et al. Posttraumatic stress symptoms related to community violence and children's diurnal cortisol response in an urban community-dwelling sample. Int J Behav Med 2009;17(1):43–50.

100. Spangler G. The emergence of adrenocortical circadian function in newborns and infants and its relationship to sleep, feeding, and maternal adrenocortical activity. Early Hum Dev 1991;25:197–208.

101. Saridjan NS, Huizink AC, Koetsier JA, et al. Do social disadvantage and early family adversity affect the diurnal cortisol rhythm in infants? The Generation R Study. Horm Behav 2010;57(2):247–54.

102. de Weerth C, van Geert P. A longitudinal study of basal cortisol in infants: intraindividual variability, circadian rhythm and developmental trends. Infant Behav Dev 2002;25:375–98.

103. Watamura SE, Donzella B, Kertes DA, et al. Developmental changes in baseline cortisol activity in early childhood: relations with napping and effortful control. Dev Psychobiol 2004;45:125–33.
104. van Cauter E, Leproult R, Kupfer DJ. Effects of gender and age on the levels and circadian rhythmicity of plasma cortisol. J Clin Endocrinol Metab 1996;81:2468–73.
105. Van Ryzin MJ, Chatham M, Kryzer E, et al. Identifying atypical cortisol patterns in young children: the benefits of group-based trajectory modeling. Psychoneuroendocrinology 2009;34:50–61.
106. Yehuda R. Biology of posttraumatic stress disorder. J Clin Psychiatry 2001;62: 41–6.
107. Pluess M, Bolten M, Pirke KM, et al. Maternal trait anxiety, emotional distress, and salivary cortisol in pregnancy. Biol Psychol 2010;83(3):169–75.
108. Harville EW, Savitz DA, Dole N, et al. Patterns of salivary cortisol secretion in pregnancy and implications for assessment protocols. Biol Psychiatry 2007; 74:85–91.
109. Jones NM, Holzman CB, Zanella AJ, et al. Assessing mid-trimester salivary cortisol levels across three consecutive days in pregnant women using an at-home collection protocol. Paediatr Perinat Epidemiol 2006;20:425–37.
110. Fox NA. Temperament and regulation of emotion in the first years of life. Pediatrics 1998;102:1230–5.
111. Card JP, Levitt P, Gluhovsky M, et al. Early experience modifies the postnatal assembly of autonomic emotional motor circuits in rats. J Neurosci 2005;25:9102–11.
112. Jansson T, Lambert GW. Effect of intrauterine growth restriction on blood pressure, glucose tolerance and sympathetic nervous system activity in the rat at 3–4 months of age. J Hypertens 1999;17:1239–48.
113. Pryce CR, Ruedi-Bettschen D, Dettling AC, et al. Early life stress: long-term physiological impact in rodents and primates. News Physiol Sci 2002;17:150–5.
114. Herlenius E, Lagercrantz H. Development of neurotransmitter systems during critical periods. Exp Neurol 2004;190:S8–21.
115. Tracey KJ. Physiology and immunology of the cholinergic antiinflammatory pathway. J Clin Invest 2007;117:289–96.
116. Sternberg EM. Neuroendocrine regulation of autoimmune/inflammatory disease. J Endocrinol 2001;169:429–35.
117. Sternberg EM. Neural regulation of innate immunity: a coordinated nonspecific host response to pathogens. Nat Rev Immunol 2006;6:318–28.
118. Carroll JL. Developmental plasticity in respiratory control. J Appl Phys 2003;94: 375–89.
119. Eckberg DL. The human respiratory gate. J Physiol 2003;548:339–52.
120. Bavis RW, Mitchell GS. Long-term effects of the perinatal environment on respiratory control. J Appl Physiol 2008;104:1220–9.
121. Alkon A, Lippert S, Vujan N, et al. The ontogeny of autonomic measures in 6- and 12-month-old infants. Dev Psychobiol 2006;48:197–208.
122. Suglia SF, Staudenmayer J, Cohen S, et al. Cumulative stress and cortisol disruption among black and Hispanic pregnant women in an urban cohort. Psychol Trauma, in press.
123. Bosquet-Enlow M, Kullowatz A, Staudenmayer J, et al. Associations of maternal lifetime trauma and perinatal traumatic stress symptoms with infant cardiorespiratory reactivity to psychological challenge. Psychosom Med 2009;71:607–14.
124. Nogueira PJ, Ferreira HH, Antunes E, et al. Chronic mild prenatal stress exacerbates the allergen-induced airway inflammation in rats. Mediators Inflamm 1999; 8:119–22.

125. Quarcoo D, Pavlovic S, Joachim RA. Stress and airway reactivity in a murine model of allergic airway inflammation. Neuroimmunomodulation 2009;16:318–24.
126. Datti F, Datti M, Antunes E, et al. Influence of chronic unpredictable stress on the allergic responses in rats. Physiol Behav 2002;77:79–83.
127. Forsythe P, Ebeling C, Gordon JR, et al. Opposing effects of short- and long-term stress on airway inflammation. Am J Respir Crit Care Med 2004;169: 220–6.
128. Joachim RA, Quarcoo D, Arck PC, et al. Stress enhances airway reactivity and airway inflammation in an animal model of allergic bronchial asthma. Psychosom Med 2003;65:811–5.
129. Joachim RA, Sagach V, Quarcoo D, et al. Neurokinin-1 receptor mediates stress-exacerbated allergic airway inflammation and airway hyperresponsiveness in mice. Psychosom Med 2004;66:564–71.
130. Okuyama K, Ohwada K, Sakurada S, et al. The distinctive effects of acute and chronic psychological stress on airway inflammation in a murine model of allergic asthma. Allergol Int 2007;56:29–35.
131. McFadden ER, Luparello T, Lyons HA, et al. The mechanism of action of suggestion in the induction of acute asthma attacks. Psychosom Med 1969;31:134–43.
132. Neild JE, Cameron IR. Bronchoconstriction in response to suggestion: its prevention by an inhaled anticholinergic agent. Br Med J 1985;290:674.
133. Ritz T, Kullowatz A. Effects of stress and emotion on lung function in health and asthma. Curr Respir Med Rev 2005;1:208–19.
134. Kullowatz A, Smith HJ, Weber S, et al. The role of the cholinergic pathway in airway response to emotional stimuli. Psychophysiology 2007;44:S71.
135. Ritz T, Thoens M, Dahme B. Modulation of respiratory sinus arrhythmia by respiration rate and volume: stability across postures and volume variations. Psychophysiology 2001;38:858–62.
136. Ritz T, Thoens M, Fahrenkrug S, et al. The airways, respiration, and respiratory sinus arrhythmia during picture viewing. Psychophysiology 2005;42:568–78.
137. Bauer AM, Quas JA, Boyce WT. Associations between physiological reactivity and children's behavior: advantages of a multisystem approach. J Dev Behav Pediatr 2002;23:102–13.
138. El-Sheikh M, Erath SA, Buckhalt JA, et al. Cortisol and children's adjustment: the moderating role of sympathetic nervous system activity. J Abnorm Child Psychol 2008;36:601–11.
139. Smeets T. Autonomic and hypothalamic-pituitary-adrenal stress resilience: impact of cardiac vagal tone. Biol Psychol 2010;84:290–5.
140. Steckler T. The molecular neurobiology of stress – evidence from genetic and epigenetic models. Behav Pharmacol 2001;12:381–427.
141. Mann JJ, Currier DM. Stress, genetics and epigenetic effects on the neurobiology of suicidal behavior and depression. Eur Psychiatry 2010;25:268–71.
142. Gilliland FD, Li YF, Saxon A, et al. Effect of glutathione-S-transferase M1 and P1 genotypes on xenobiotic enhancement of allergic responses: randomised, placebo-controlled crossover study. Lancet 2004;10(363):119–25.
143. Child F, Lenney W, Clayton S, et al. The association of maternal but not paternal genetic variation in GSTP1 with asthma phenotypes in children. Respir Med 2003;97:1247–56.
144. Wust S, Van Rossum EF, Federenko IS, et al. Common polymorphisms in the glucocorticoid receptor gene are associated with adrenocortical responses to psychosocial stress. J Clin Endocrinol Metab 2004;89:565–73.

145. Yamada Y, Nakamura H, Adachi T, et al. Elevated serum levels of thioredoxin in patients with acute exacerbation of asthma. Immunol Lett 2003;86:199–205.
146. Uhart M, McCaul ME, Oswald LM, et al. GABRA6 gene polymorphism and an attenuated stress response. Mol Psychiatry 2004;9(11):998–1006.
147. Jeanmonod P, von Kanel R, Maly FE, et al. Elevated plasma C-reactive protein in chronically distressed subjects who carry the A allele of the TNF-alpha -308 G/A polymorphism. Psychosom Med 2004;66:501–6.
148. Jaenisch R, Bird A. Epigenetic regulation of gene expression: how the genome integrates intrinsic and environmental signals. Nat Genet 2003;35:245–54.
149. Miller RL, Ho SM. Environmental epigenetics and asthma: current concepts and call for studies. Am J Respir Crit Care Med 2008;177:567–73.
150. Prescott SL, Clifton V. Asthma and pregnancy: emerging evidence of epigenetic interactions in utero. Curr Opin Allergy Clin Immunol 2009;9:417–26.
151. Castro M, Ramirez MI, Gern JE, et al. Strategic plan for pediatric respiratory diseases research: an NHLBI working group report. Proc Am Thorac Soc 2009;15:1–10.
152. Levenson JM, Sweatt JD. Epigenetic mechanisms: a common theme in vertebrate and invertebrate memory formation. Cell Mol Life Sci 2006;63:1009–16.
153. Miller GE, Chen E, Zhou ES. If it goes up, must it come down? Chronic stress and the hypothalamic-pituitary-adrenal axis in humans. Psychol Bull 2007;133:25–45.
154. Meaney MJ, Szyf M. Maternal care as a model for experience-dependent chromatin plasticity? Trends Neurosci 2005;28:456–63.
155. Szyf M, McGowan P, Meaney MJ. The social environment and the epigenome. Environ Mol Mutagen 2008;49:46–60.
156. Turner JD, Pelascini LP, Macedo JA, et al. Highly individual methylation patterns of alternative glucocorticoid receptor promoters suggest individualized epigenetic regulatory mechanisms. Nucleic Acids Res 2008;36:7207–18.
157. Krozowski ZS, Provencher PH, Smith RE, et al. Isozymes of 11 beta-hydroxysteroid dehydrogenase: which enzyme endows mineralocorticoid specificity? Steroids 1994;59:116–20.
158. Esposito E, Cuzzocrea S. The role of nitric oxide synthases in lung inflammtion. Curr Opin Investig Drugs 2007;8:899–909.
159. Danson EJ, Li D, Wang I, et al. Targeting cardiac sympatho-vagal imbalance using gene transfer of nitric oxide synthase. J Mol Cell Cardiol 2009;46:482–9.
160. McLeod TM, Lopez-Figueroa AL, Lopez-Figueroa MO. Nitric oxide, stress, and depression. Psychopharmacol Bull 2001;35:24–41.
161. Tarantini L, Bonzini M, Apostoli P, et al. Effects of particulate matter on genomic DNA methylation content and iNOS promoter methylation. Environ Health Perspect 2009;117:217–22.
162. Alikhani-Koopaei R, Fouladkou F, Frey FJ, et al. Epigenetic regulation of 11 beta-hydroxysteroid dehydrogenase type 2 expression. J Clin Invest 2004;114:1146–57.
163. Weaver IC, Cervoni N, Champagne FA, et al. Epigenetic programming by maternal behavior. Nat Neurosci 2004;7:847–54.
164. McGowan PO, Sasaki A, D'Alessio AC, et al. Epigenetic regulation of the glucocorticoid receptor in human brain associated with childhood abuse. Nat Neurosci 2009;12:342–8.
165. Oberlander TF, Weinberg J, Papsdorf M, et al. Prenatal exposure to maternal depression, neonatal methylation of human glucocorticoid receptor gene (NR3C1) and infant cortisol stress responses. Epigenetics 2008;3:97–106.

166. Stokols D. Establishing and maintaining healthy environments: toward a social ecology of health promotion. Am Psychol 1992;47:6–22.
167. Francis DD. Conceptualizing child health disparities: a role for developmental neurogenomics. Pediatrics 2009;124:S196–202.
168. Wright RJ, Subramanian SV. Advancing a multilevel framework for epidemiological research on asthma disparities. Chest 2007;132:757S–69S.
169. Evans G. Environmental stress and health. In: Baum A, Revenson T, Singer J, editors. Handbook of health psychology. Mahwah (NJ): Lawrence Erlbaum; 2001. p. 365–85.
170. Williams DR, Sternthal M, Wright RJ. Social determinants: taking the social context of asthma seriously. Pediatrics 2009;3:S174–84.
171. Braveman P, Marchi K, Egerter S, et al. Poverty, near-poverty, and hardship around the time of pregnancy. Matern Child Health J 2010;14(1):20–35.
172. Kessler RC, Sonnega A, Bromet E, et al. Posttraumatic stress disorder in the national comorbidity survey. Arch Gen Psychiatry 1995;52:1048–60.
173. Holman EA, Silver RC, Waitzkin H. Traumatic life events in primary care patients: a study in an ethnically diverse sample. Arch Fam Med 2000;9:802–10.
174. Hien D, Bukszpan C. Interpersonal violence in a "normal" low-income control group. Womens Health 1999;29:1–16.
175. Clark C, Ryan L, Kawachi I, et al. Witnessing community violence in residential neighborhoods: a mental health hazard for urban women. J Urban Health 2007; 85:22–38.
176. Brown JR, Hill HM, Lambert SF. Traumatic stress symptoms in women exposed to community and partner violence. J Interpers Violence 2005;20:1478–94.
177. Sternthal MJ, Bosquet Enlow M, Cohen S, et al. Maternal interpersonal trauma and cord blood IgE levels in an inner-city cohort: a life-course perspective. J Allergy Clin Immunol 2009;124:954–60.
178. Sternthal MJ, Hun HJ, Earls F, et al. Community violence and urban childhood asthma: a multilevel analysis. Eur Respir J 2010. [Epub ahead of print].
179. Sandel M, Wright RJ. Expanding dimensions of housing that influence asthma morbidity: when home is where the stress is. Arch Dis Child 2006;91:942–8.
180. Quinn K, Kaufman JS, Siddiqi A, et al. Stress and the city: housing stressors are associated with respiratory health among low socioeconomic status Chicago children. J Urban Health 2010;87(4):688–702.
181. Mrazek DA, Klinnert M, Mrazek PJ, et al. Prediction of early-onset asthma in genetically at-risk children. Pediatr Pulmonol 1999;27:85–94.
182. Wright RJ, Cohen S, Carey V, et al. Parental stress as a predictor of wheezing in infancy: a prospective birth-cohort study. Am J Respir Crit Care Med 2002;165: 358–65.
183. Clougherty J, Levy JI, Kubzansky LD, et al. The effects of traffic-related air pollution and exposure to violence on urban asthma etiology. Environ Health Perspect 2007;115:1140–6.
184. Chen E, Schreier HM, Strunk RC, et al. Chronic traffic-related air pollution and stress interact to predict biologic and clinical outcomes in asthma. Environ Health Perspect 2008;116:970–5.
185. Shankardass K, McConnell R, Jerrett M, et al. Parental stress increases the effect of traffic-related air pollution on childhood asthma incidence. Proc Natl Acad Sci U S A 2009;106:12406–11.

Clinical Potentials for Measuring Stress in Youth with Asthma

Hannah M.C. Schreier, MA*, Gregory E. Miller, PhD,
Edith Chen, PhD

KEYWORDS

• Psychological stress • Asthma • Measurement

STRESS AND ASTHMA

It has long been recognized by clinicians and researchers that asthma can be affected by numerous triggers in the physical environment. Among the best understood contributors to asthma are environmental pollutants,[1] such as exposure to traffic-related air pollution[2] and indoor exposure to a variety of allergens[3] and environmental tobacco smoke.[4,5] Similarly, viral infections of the upper and lower respiratory tracts have been linked to asthmatic symptoms.[6]

More recently, increasing attention has focused on the contribution of potential triggers from the social environment, such as stressors.[7] Psychological stress has been increasingly implicated in pediatric asthma[8] and linked to many clinical asthma outcomes, including physician visits and hospitalizations.[9] Several studies provide intriguing evidence of the potential influence that psychosocial stressors can have on asthma outcomes. Several case studies suggest the onset and worsening of asthma symptoms among youth shortly after they themselves or people close to them have experienced negative life events.[10] These negative life events included being the victim of acts of violence or witnessing violent acts, as well as witnessing severe conflict among parents; in all cases, youth experienced significant, acute episodes of asthma. Also of interest is the observation that in some cases the fluctuations in asthma exacerbations changed hand in hand with the presence or absence of psychosocial stressors in the environment, for example the known presence of one's assailant in the neighborhood.

Additional evidence comes from a prospective, longitudinal study which followed 6- to 13-year-old children with asthma for 18 months and involved repeated assessments of life stress through interviews and the collection of daily diary and peak flow

This work was supported by NIH grant HL073975 and the William T. Grant Foundation.
Department of Psychology, University of British Columbia, 2136 West Mall, Vancouver, BC V6T 1Z4, Canada
* Corresponding author.
E-mail address: hannahs@psych.ubc.ca

Immunol Allergy Clin N Am 31 (2011) 41–54
doi:10.1016/j.iac.2010.09.003
0889-8561/11/$ – see front matter © 2011 Elsevier Inc. All rights reserved.
immunology.theclinics.com

information.[11] In this study, youth were significantly more likely to experience new asthma attacks in the weeks following negative life events, such as the death of a close person. These effects were even more pronounced among youth whom interviews revealed to experience chronic stress in other areas of their lives, for example being bullied at school or coming from a conflictual home environment.

Hence, although several psychological factors are believed to be related to pediatric asthma outcomes,[12] the influence of psychological stress has been of particular interest, especially because it may exacerbate other psychological problems, including anxiety and depression. One way in which psychological stress may exert its effects is by moderating and potentiating the effects of physical environmental triggers, making individuals more vulnerable to these triggers.

There are numerous ways of measuring stress in people's lives. Researchers use a variety of measures ranging from the administration of self-report questionnaires to the assessment of life events through in-depth interviews. This article differentiates between various conceptualizations of stress and the measurement approaches that are associated with them; provides an overview of the most widely used methods for assessing stress among patients with asthma and discusses their strengths and weaknesses; and reviews evidence for how well different measures of stress can be linked to clinical outcomes and the biologic processes that underlie them.

WHAT IS STRESS?

Stress has been conceptualized in many different ways.[13] Among the most common views of stress are the environmental and the subjective perspectives, which also map onto the different measurement strategies used in today's research. The environmental stress perspective focuses on external demands that individuals encounter as part of their life experience.[14] These demands come in the form of stressors that the individual has to manage, and the assumption is that they will have a fairly uniform effect on people's health,[15] determined by how much change or adaptation is required.

In contrast, there has been an alternative conceptualization of stress that focuses on the interaction of the person and the demands being faced.[16] This view focuses on how people interpret or appraise a stressor, in terms of whether it poses a threat to their goals, and whether they are able to cope with it effectively. The assumption here is that not all events are perceived in the same way by all people, and that only those that are appraised as stressful (ie, threatening and unmanageable) will ultimately prove to be detrimental to health.[17] Thus, although one person may experience a transition to a new work environment as a considerable stressor, it may be unmemorable to another person. This view highlights the importance of assessing subjective perceptions of events and people's beliefs as to whether they think they will be able to successfully cope with the stressor at hand.

The currently used measurement approaches tend to reflect one tradition or the other. Life-event checklists that assess and sum the number of life events a person has experienced within a certain time frame follow from an environmental stress perspective. Other approaches that are more focused on investigating a person's experience of life events, for example by asking people to complete questionnaires about what kind of effect an event has had on their life, are closer to focusing on subjective stress appraisals.

Aside from differentiating the objective occurrence of events from the subjective experience of an event, researchers also make distinctions regarding the nature of the event itself. For example, some stressors are distinct and time limited (acute stressors), whereas others are long lasting and without definitive endpoints[18] (chronic stress). Acute stressors can be further divided into major life events (eg, being in a car accident) and smaller acute stressors akin to daily hassles (eg, dealing with traffic when commuting to work).[19] There are also stressors that blur the distinction between acute and chronic (eg, a brief event such as a natural disaster, which triggers a string of other challenges such as repairing one's home, finding the money to do so, and so forth). Thus, stressors will vary in both intensity and duration, and it is important to consider these dimensions in measuring stress, because they may have different effects on asthma outcomes.

This article first reviews the evidence for the influence of stress on clinical asthma outcomes and the biologic mechanisms that are believed to mediate these relationships, before addressing the different ways of assessing stress.

EVIDENCE FOR A LINK BETWEEN STRESS AND ASTHMA

Research to date, implementing different methods of stress measurement, suggests a clear relationship between stress and both the onset[20] and course of asthma.[8,21] For example, using a life-event checklist the onset of asthma has been associated with retrospective recall of greater life stressors in the years preceding and concurrent to asthma diagnosis among a sample of university students.[22] Interview-based assessments of adolescents' stress perceptions, including acute and chronic stressors as well as subjective stress interpretations, were found to be associated with patterns of immune response known to be involved in the worsening of asthma, including greater in vitro mitogen-stimulated production of the cytokines interleukin 5 (IL-5) and interferon-γ (IFN-γ).[23] Youth from more stable home environments (ie, youth of parents who reported less parenting stress on a self-report questionnaire) seem to be exposed to more routines at home, which in turn is associated with improved medication adherence.[24]

Other approaches, including experimental manipulations of stress, further underscore the influence of psychosocial stressors on airway functioning. In one study, a group of older children and adolescents asked to relate an embarrassing story to a tape recorder in the presence of an adult experimenter subsequently showed evidence of greater airway resistance.[25] In a small sample of adults with asthma, everyday stressors assessed across a 10-day period using preprogrammed watches, were linked to participants' peak expiratory flow rate (PEFR) as well as asthma symptoms.[26] Hence, connections between psychosocial stress and clinical asthma outcomes have been shown using different research methodologies and study designs.

BIOLOGIC MECHANISMS LINKING STRESS AND ASTHMA

Why would psychological stress be linked to the onset and course of asthma? Asthma is a disease that involves excessive airway inflammatory responses to environmental triggers, such as allergens and pollution.[27] Thus, one model posits that psychological stress accentuates the magnitude of inflammatory responses to these triggers. Specifically, many indoor and outdoor triggers have been linked to asthma exacerbations. For example, living in greater proximity to traffic has been associated with asthma outcomes[28] among youth, likely as a result of the increased exposure to traffic-related pollution that is also known to negatively influence asthma.[29–31] Within their home environments, youth are exposed to other environmental triggers that are associated with worsened asthma. Among the most common triggers are exposure to environmental tobacco smoke, which has been shown to lead to more emergency department visits among youth,[5] and indoor allergens, such as mouse and cockroach allergens, which result in greater asthma morbidity.[3,32]

The inflammatory pathway that becomes activated in response to these environmental stimuli and leads to asthma involves the activation of T helper cells. On exposure to allergens, pathogens, and some irritants, dendritic cells present fragments of these triggers to T helper cells, which then coordinate downstream immunologic responses that drive the pathophysiology of asthma episodes. Distinctions are often made between 2 classes of T helper cells, Th1 and Th2 cells, which are functionally, but not morphologically, different. Specifically, Th1 cells are involved primarily in cell-mediated immunity and produce cytokines such as IFN-γ. In contrast, Th2 cells coordinate a humoral, or antibody-mediated, response to allergen exposure. Asthma is often believed to be marked by a shift toward Th2-dependent processes, as mediated through 2 main pathways, an early-phase response involving IL-4 and IL-13 and late-phase response involving IL-5.[33]

Th2 cells release IL-4 and IL-13,[34] which promote the proliferation and differentiation of B cells. B cells then synthesize and release immunoglobulin E antibodies that bind to mast cells in the airways, causing them to degranulate and release allergic mediators such as histamines and leukotrienes. These mediators induce smooth muscle constriction, mucus production, and edema, resulting in early-phase asthma symptoms. An alternative pathway involves the release of IL-5 by Th2 cells.[35] IL-5 is partly responsible for the production, maturation, and activation of eosinophils. Once they are recruited to the airways, eosinophils result in both greater inflammation and airway obstruction. Eosinophils release other mediators, for example eosinophil cationic protein, which can damage airway cells, and leukotrienes, which cause edema and further bronchial construction. Hence, this second pathway through IL-5 and eosinophils is believed to be involved in the more chronic, long-term inflammation associated with asthma. For more in-depth discussions of psychological stress and its effects on inflammation and asthma exacerbations, as well as more information on inflammation in asthma in general, see the brief reviews by Chen and Miller[27] and Busse and Lemanske.[36]

Several studies support the importance of assessing these biologic indicators and have linked stress to these processes. Research from our laboratory has shown that, among youth with asthma, greater chronic family stress is associated with greater in vitro stimulated production of cytokines implicated in asthma, including IL-5 and IL-13, as well as in vivo mobilization and activation of eosinophils.[37,38] Similarly, studies have found that examination-related stress potentiates IL-5 production and eosinophil mobilization in sputum following an airway challenge,[39] as well as decreased natural killer cell cytotoxicity[40] among university students with asthma.

MEASURING STRESS

There follows a discussion of the most common approaches to measuring stress, their benefits and disadvantages, and how they relate to asthma-relevant outcomes.

Experimental and Quasi-experimental Approaches

Laboratory manipulations

Some researchers have taken advantage of the controlled laboratory environment to assess the influence of various stressors on asthma-related outcomes that can be closely monitored before, during, and following exposure to psychological stressors. Laboratory manipulations frequently involve participants completing tasks, such as public speaking, engaging in discussions, or watching stressful movies. This approach has the advantage that researchers can easily compare changes in the outcome variable of interest from before to after stressor exposure, or between groups who have or have not been exposed. Assuming the subjects have been randomly assigned in sufficient numbers to stressor versus control conditions, the researcher can make causal inferences about the influence of the manipulation, without concerns about confounding variables playing a role.

One laboratory manipulation suggests that emotional responsivity may mediate the relationship between psychological stress and asthma outcomes.[41] As part of this study, youth with asthma watched several segments from the movie, *E.T., The Extra-terrestrial*. Youth who had stronger emotional responses to these movie segments exhibited increased airway reactivity and decreased pulmonary functioning, as measured by youth's forced expiratory volume in 1 second (FEV_1). Similarly, youth with asthma who underwent a stressful task in the laboratory, relating an embarrassing moment to a tape recorder in the presence of an adult experimenter, exhibited decreased airway resistance following this task.[25] Furthermore, among adolescents with asthma, exposure to a stressful computer task was sufficient to induce breathlessness, even in the absence of actual airway obstruction.[42]

Research from our own laboratory has also investigated the effects of stress on markers of airway inflammation among healthy youth and youth with asthma using an acute stress task in the laboratory.[43] Youth and their parents were asked to discuss a topic of disagreement for 8 minutes, and youth's airway inflammation was assessed using a measure of exhaled nitric oxide both before and after the acute stress task. Increases in youth's heart rate and blood pressure indicated that youth did experience these discussions as stressful. In addition, youth with asthma, but not healthy youth, also experienced changes in their levels of exhaled nitric oxide, depending on the socioeconomic status (SES) of their background. Youth from low-SES families experienced increases in exhaled nitric oxide about 45 minutes after participating in the acute stress task, whereas youth from high-SES families experienced decreases, indicating that acute psychosocial stressors affect airway inflammation and that this response is moderated by SES.

Naturally occurring stressors

Some studies take advantage of naturally occurring stressors to assess the influence of psychological stress on asthma. Although this does not give experimenters the same amount of experimental control, or the ability to make causal inferences, it has the advantage of greater ecological validity because participants are experiencing stressors outside the artificial laboratory environment.

Commonly used paradigms involving naturally occurring stressors include examination stress among students. Liu and colleagues[39] asked college students with mild allergic asthma to undergo an inhaled antigen challenge at 2 separate time points, once during a low-stress midsemester time point and once during final examination week; that is, during a more stressful time. The inhaled antigen challenge involved the administration of increasingly high doses of allergens to which the participants were sensitized (eg, dust mite or cat dander) until their lung functioning had declined by 20% or more. During the high-stress final examination period, the inhaled antigen challenge resulted in a greater sputum eosinophil response as well as a greater decrease in FEV_1 from before to after the challenge. These results suggest that naturally occurring stressors amplify the inflammatory response to asthma triggers, and therefore have the potential to worsen clinical outcomes.

Some researchers are assessing naturally occurring stressors on an ongoing daily basis; that is, how the small stressors to which people are exposed in their everyday lives may influence their health. The preferred way for studying stress in everyday life is through a daily diary.[44] By asking participants to briefly report on the stressors they experienced throughout a given day, every evening or multiple times throughout the day, researchers can link the stressors to health outcomes.

One study investigating the effects of daily psychological stress among adults with asthma asked participants to complete 5 daily diary assessments a day, for 10 days.[26] Participants were beeped at random times throughout the day, asked about the occurrence of stressful life events, and asked to complete a peak flow reading. Results suggested that there were diurnal patterns to asthma symptoms and PEFR and that these could be accounted for by psychosocial factors, including stressors. Experiencing more stressors was associated with lower PEFR and more asthma symptoms. Hence, daily diary assessments of stress may prove valuable for understanding the influence of everyday stressors on lung function and asthma outcomes.

Advantages and disadvantages

Experimental manipulations are beneficial in that they allow researchers to fully control the environment in which stressors occur, thereby ensuring that observed changes in asthma outcomes can be attributed to stressor exposure. In addition, assessing asthma outcomes in response to psychological stressors in the laboratory enables researchers to assess changes via objective markers, rather than having to rely on participant-reported outcomes, such as symptoms, or other clinical outcomes, such as emergency department visits. The primary criticism of laboratory manipulations relates to the questionable extent to which stress responses experienced in the laboratory can be generalized to real-life situations. However, to the extent that experimental manipulations are representative of real-life stressors, the controlled laboratory environments can provide important information regarding how stressors result in physiologic changes that ultimately lead to increased asthma morbidity. Taking advantage of naturally occurring stressors results in greater ecological validity but decreases the amount of control and inferential leverage researchers have.

Furthermore, a daily diary approach allows for more frequent data collection that is less likely to be affected by participants' recall bias. However, daily diaries can be disruptive to people's lives and require a significant amount of effort from participants, and hence information is typically only collected for brief periods of time (eg, 2 weeks) during which participants may not experience many life stressors. However, depending on the study design, it may be possible to integrate several periods of daily diary data collection into a longitudinal study design and ask participants to complete multiple rounds of daily diary, several weeks or months apart.

Environmental Occurrence of Stressors and Life-Event Checklists

An alternative approach is to assess the types of stressors that are occurring in individuals' lives. For example, life-event checklists consist of lists of events that are experienced by the general population and believed to be experienced as stressful by most people, such as moving to a new place, getting divorced, or starting a new job. Participants simply check all the items on a particular life-event checklist that they have experienced within a given time frame, for example, the last 30 days. Researchers can then sum the number of items checked and use the total score as an indicator of the amount of stress in an individual's life. For an overview of existing checklists see Turner and Wheaton.[45]

Turyk and colleagues[9] used a 15-item checklist to assess the effect of stressful life events believed to commonly occur among inner-city youth with and without asthma. Although asthma morbidity was generally high in this sample, the number of stressful life events youth reported having been exposed to in the past year was associated with asthma symptoms, missed school days, physician contact, and hospitalization for asthma. In addition, the investigators found a dose-response relationship between the number of stressful life experiences and the odds of dry cough at night, number of symptoms, and physician visits for asthma, such that experiencing increasing numbers of negative life events was related to a greater number of symptoms and physician visits. These results remained significant even after several potentially relevant confounding variables were taken into account.

Advantages and disadvantages

Life-event checklists have clear advantages in that they are quick and cheap to administer and do not require any training on the part of the research team. Hence, they may be particularly useful in large samples or when time for stress assessments is limited (eg, in epidemiologic studies). However, although checklists are easy to use, the information that can be collected through them is limited. For example, the events on a checklist may not be a good representation of events experienced by people in the population of interest. Hence, events may be missed entirely if stressful events that participants considered important were not part of a checklist. Alternatively, participants may decline to report an event that has occurred, either because they do not want to disclose them, or they believe they were not of sufficient importance to merit doing so. In addition, these types of self-reports usually do not assess the specific timing or duration of events and fail to capture the participants' appraisal of an event. For example, participants may select items on a checklist because they have experienced them even if they did not consider the occurrence of such an event stressful. As a result, some people consider checklists a better measure of the change occurring in people's lives, rather than negative life events or stress per se.[45]

Assessing Subjective Stress Appraisal

Another common approach to assessing stress in the literature involves self-report questionnaires regarding subjective perceptions of stress in individuals' lives. The Perceived Stress Scale (PSS),[46] for example, is a frequently used 10-item measure that assesses subjective stress experiences by asking participants how stressful they consider their life is in general; for example, how unpredictable they find it to be. Most self-report questionnaires require participants to indicate to what extent they endorse statements assessing their subjective stress experiences on Likert scales; that is, indicating the extent to which they agree or disagree with certain statements on a scale ranging from 5 to 7. These responses can then be summed to create a total score representative of the amount of stress subjectively experienced by participants.

One study has used the PSS to assess stress among caregivers of youth predisposed to atopy throughout early life.[47] Caregivers repeatedly completed the PSS, and results indicated that youth whose parents reported greater perceived stress showed evidence, at the age of 2 to 3 years, of greater IgE expression, a greater allergen-induced proliferative response, as well as changes in cytokine production indicating increased airway inflammation. This study suggests that data gained from questionnaire-based stress assessments among caregivers are relevant regarding the overall immunologic profiles of youth at risk for asthma.

However, another study that assessed the influence of social support among college students with asthma on their immune functioning during low-stress (midsemester) and, presumably, high-stress (final examination period) times found that, although students experienced physiologic changes between midsemester and the final examination period, they did not report higher levels of stress during the examination period. This suggests that some questionnaire-based assessments of subjective stress experiences may be insensitive to certain types of stressors or among particular populations.[40]

An alternative approach to assessing subjective appraisals involves a controlled laboratory presentation of a life event, from which individual perceptions of that event can then be assessed. The Cognitive Appraisal and Understanding of Social Events (CAUSE) videos[48] were developed to assess people's interpretation of events that have ambiguous outcomes. For example, one of these videos depicts a high school girl browsing in a department store with an overly attentive saleswoman nearby. Participants are asked to imagine themselves in the place of the teenager when watching the video and are subsequently asked about their interpretation of the situation (eg, "Why do you think the saleswoman was paying attention to you while you were browsing?"). By asking participants about their appraisal of this potentially stressful situation, one can code their responses to these ambiguous situations as being more benign (eg, she was trying to make a sale) or hostile (eg, she believed I was about to steal something).

Research from our laboratory using the CAUSE videos indicates that, as with chronic stress, participants' perceived threat in response to an ambiguous social situation also predicts a heightened inflammatory profile (specifically, increased stimulated IL-5 and IL-13 production) as well as higher eosinophil counts among youth with asthma.[37] In addition, other studies found stress interpretations to statistically mediate the relationship between low SES and greater stimulated cytokine production in adolescents with asthma[23] and between low SES and gene transcription control pathways regulating inflammation and catecholamine signaling in adolescents with asthma.[49]

Advantages and disadvantages

Similar to life-event checklists, assessments of subjective stress appraisals are easy to administer and require little time and effort. They also address what some researchers conceptualize as the essence of the stress response: the subjective perception of stress.

However, this reliance on the subjective can create certain measurement problems. For example, people may differ in their subjective assessments of situations and assess stressful life events according to idiosyncratic standards. As a result, it can be difficult to know whether individual differences in responding reflect variations in the occurrence versus the perception of an event. It is also possible that people use scales differently when making ratings, or that they are unwilling to relate details of events that they perceived to be embarrassing, hence rating an event as less severe or important than it may have been. In addition, because different people use different, subjective reference points when making ratings of the effects of stressful life events, meaningful comparisons across individuals may be difficult, if not impossible. Consequently, such an approach may be more useful when investigating within-person changes across several time points.

Interviews

Many studies interested in assessing the influence of psychological stress on asthma also do so through interviews, such as the UCLA Life Stress Interview (LSI)[50] and the Life Events and Difficulties Schedule.[51] These interviews probe both the occurrence of ongoing difficulties (chronic stress) across several life domains, such as family, friends, and school/work, as well as the occurrence of time-limited events that are typically short in duration (acute events). Ratings of the severity of acute and chronic stress are made by interviewers (rather than by the participants themselves) and typically take into account context. For example, chronic stress may be rated on a 1 to 5 scale for each domain of interest by the interviewer, with higher numbers reflecting more severe difficulties. In addition, acute stressors and their objective effects may be rated by a team of interviewers. Interviewers are briefed on the details about a given event and subsequently agree on a consensus rating, also on a 5-point scale, taking into account the context of a particular situation, such as whether an event was expected and whether a similar event had previously taken place.

Several studies have successfully implemented interview-based approaches to measuring stress and linked them to outcomes relevant to asthma. Studies from our own research group have repeatedly used the LSI.[52] Using this approach, we have linked stress in the lives of youth with asthma to various biologic outcomes. Specifically, we have investigated the effects of stress in vitro by culturing peripheral mononuclear blood cells with a mitogen cocktail consisting of phorbol myristate acetate and ionomycin and subsequently measuring the amount of cytokines being produced. We have found that, among youth with asthma between the ages of 9 and 18 years, greater chronic home and family stress was associated with an increased production of IL-5, IL-13, and higher levels of circulating eosinophils, whereas the opposite was true for a healthy comparison group.[37] We have also linked greater home life stress among youth with asthma to a decreased output of salivary α-amylase across the day,[53] indicating lower sympathetic activity. This finding suggests another possible mechanism through which stress in the lives of youth with asthma may lead to asthma exacerbations.

Chen and colleagues[54] also found interactions of interview-based stress measures with physical environment measures of air pollution in predicting asthma outcomes. Specifically, higher levels of chronic family stress were associated with higher IL-5 production, IgE levels, and eosinophil counts among youth with asthma living in neighborhoods with modest levels of traffic-related air pollution. In contrast, among youth living in neighborhoods with high traffic-related pollution, psychological stress was not associated with inflammatory profiles. These interaction effects also extended to clinical changes over 6 months, such that, among youth with asthma living in neighborhoods with modest levels of traffic-related air pollution, higher levels of chronic family stress predicted increases in asthma symptoms and declines in pulmonary function in a 6-month follow-up period. These findings suggest that, when physical environment exposures are modest, social environment exposures may exert their greatest effects, whereas high levels of physical environment exposures may overwhelm effects of the social environment.

Other research groups have also evaluated the effects of interview-based stress on clinical asthma outcomes among youth. As part of a prospective 18-month longitudinal study, Sandberg and colleagues[55] used the Psychosocial Assessment of Childhood Experiences (PACE) interview[56] to repeatedly assess the occurrence of life events across the study period.[57] Sandberg and colleagues[55] found that the likelihood of youth experiencing a new asthma attack increased shortly after the experience of a stressful life event, and again roughly 5 to 7 weeks later.

Some measures are also beginning to circumvent the problems inherent in questionnaire and checklist approaches by supplementing the traditional checklist approach with additional questions that allow for the collection of more in-depth data. One such measure, the Crisis in Family Systems (CRISYS)[58] instrument, successfully combines quantitative and qualitative approaches. Participants first indicate, using a checklist format, whether they have experienced a particular set of stressful life events. In addition, they answer questions for items they endorsed, either on a Likert scale or in response to open-ended questions from an interviewer, and provide more detailed information about the event in question. Hence, this represents a successful combination of different approaches to stress measurement. Shalowitz and colleagues[59] used this measure to assess stress among caregivers of youth with asthma and found that children of mothers who experienced more negative life stressors were more likely to have high, rather than low or moderate, asthma morbidity.

There is also mounting evidence that chronic and acute stress need to be considered together to allow for a coherent assessment of the effects of stress on asthma outcomes. For example, Sandberg and colleagues[11] investigated the effects of chronic and acute stress among children between the ages of 6 and 13 years as part of an 18-month prospective study. Although youth who experienced an acute stress event had an increased likelihood of an asthma attack in the weeks following the event, youth who were also exposed to chronic stress showed a shortened latency to asthma exacerbations following the acute stressor.

Similarly, Marin and colleagues[60] found that youth with asthma who experienced acute stressors in the context of high chronic stress showed increased inflammatory profiles in response to stress. Youth participated in 5 study visits across 5 years (ie, once every 6 months) and, among youth living in a home environment marked by increased chronic family stress, at times when they had recently experienced an acute stressor they exhibited heightened stimulated production of asthma-relevant cytokines such as IL-4 and IL-5 compared with times when they had not recently experienced an acute stressor. In addition, youth provided information on their asthma symptoms for 2 weeks following each laboratory visit. Among those with more severe asthma, at times when participants exhibited higher levels of stimulated cytokine production, they also reported more asthma symptoms, pointing to the clinical significance of the observed changes in stimulated cytokine production.

The co-occurrence of chronic and acute life stress events among youth with asthma has been linked to gene expression profiles relevant to asthma inflammation.[61] Youth with asthma experiencing chronic stress in their homes and who also experienced a major acute life event within the previous 6 months exhibited reduced expression of glucocorticoid receptor mRNA and β2-adrenergic receptor mRNA. This reduction could potentially lead to a decreased sensitivity to the antiinflammatory properties of glucocorticoids, resulting in greater airway inflammation, as well as to a decreased efficacy of asthma medications that target these receptors. Together, these studies suggest that, when studying acute stress in particular, chronic stress should also be assessed because it may significantly moderate people's response to acute stressors.

Advantages and disadvantages

Using semistructured interviews allows researchers to use a repertoire of follow-up questions to probe for additional detail regarding stressful life events. This greater flexibility makes it possible to obtain information regarding the circumstances surrounding an event, exacerbating and mitigating factors, details about the timing and duration of the event, and the participant's appraisal of an event. In addition, semistructured interviews, as opposed to structured interviews, provide the advantage of allowing the interviewer to ask whatever questions are most relevant to a certain event and participants, instead of working with a fixed set of questions that are answered by all participants.

Other advantages of using an interview-based approach are the assessment of contextual information that can aid in making severity ratings, and having interviewers, rather than participants, making ratings of stress. Specifically, within the context of a semistructured interview, an interviewer will be able to obtain additional information on events that would not have been available through a checklist approach, for example a participant's perceived sense of ability to control an event. This information can then be used to make a more objective rating of an event by rating the normative stress levels that would commonly be associated with it. This in turn allows the researcher to distinguish between normative events (eg, child transitioned from middle to high school and is adjusting well to their new school), and more stressful events (eg, child got expelled from old school because of behavioral problems and was forced to attend a new school midsemester). Note that in both cases children may have endorsed a "Switched schools in the past half year" item on a checklist even though the exact circumstances between these situations vary widely. Although the former situation represents a normative transition, the latter does not and is likely to be associated with significantly greater stress. Within the framework of contextual interviews, researchers can make more objective ratings of the stress associated with the particular life events that participants report, rather than having to rely on participants' ratings. Having obtained all this additional information, researchers will be able to make well-informed and objective ratings of stressful life events.

Interview-based assessments that capture stress across a variety of domains also allow for comparisons of the relative effects from domain to domain. For example, across several studies from our laboratory we find that chronic stress in the family domain has robust associations with asthma inflammatory measures, but that chronic stress in other domains, such as friendship and school, are not associated with inflammatory profiles in asthma.[60–62]

Using an interview-based approach has its costs, primarily in terms of the greater burden on both the participants and researchers. Interview-based assessments of stress require training of interviewers, regular checks on inter-rater reliability, and take longer to administer than questionnaire-based assessments. Hence these approaches are more costly, labor-intensive, and may not be feasible in larger samples.

SUMMARY

This article reviews different methods of assessing stress that are most commonly being used in current research. Quicker ways of measuring stress, for example, through self-report questionnaires and event checklists, may be the necessary tools for large-scale studies and can be easily implemented. However, there are concerns regarding the quality of information that can be gained from these measures and they may not always be sensitive enough. An alternative to these measures is interview-based assessments of an individual's stress. Although they are more resource intensive, we believe that the flexibility and resulting in-depth information that can be gained from interview-based approaches are worth the increased costs in terms of time and labor, because research suggests robust associations of interview-based stress measures with both asthma biologic and clinical outcomes. Research on stress and asthma should also take into account subjective appraisals of stress, as well as dimensions such as duration and intensity in characterizing stress. Through a more sophisticated understanding of the dimensions of stress that are associated with asthma pathophysiologic processes and functional impairment, researchers and clinicians will be able to identify the components of stress that would be important to target, together with medication compliance and environmental exposures in multi-pronged behavioral interventions intended to reduce asthma morbidity.

REFERENCES

1. Nelson HS, Szefler SJ, Jacobs J, et al. The relationships among environmental allergen sensitization, allergen exposure, pulmonary function, and bronchial

hyperresponsiveness in the childhood asthma management program. J Allergy Clin Immunol 1999;104(4 Pt 1):775–85.

2. Trasande L, Thurston GD. The role of air pollution in asthma and other pediatric morbidities. J Allergy Clin Immunol 2005;115(4):689–99.

3. Lanphear BP, Kahn RS, Berger O, et al. Contribution of residential exposures to asthma in US children and adolescents. Pediatrics 2001;107(6):E98.

4. Berz JB, Carter AS, Wagmiller RL, et al. Prevalence and correlates of early onset asthma and wheezing in a healthy birth cohort of 2- to 3-year olds. J Pediatr Psychol 2007;32(2):154–66.

5. Wang HC, McGeady SJ, Yousef E. Patient, home residence, and neighborhood characteristics in pediatric emergency department visits for asthma. J Asthma 2007;44(2):95–8.

6. Sigurs N, Gustafsson PM, Bjarnason R, et al. Severe respiratory syncytial virus bronchiolitis in infancy and asthma and allergy at age 13. Am J Respir Crit Care Med 2005;171(2):137–41.

7. Chen E, Schreier HM. Does the social environment contribute to asthma? Immunol Allergy Clin North Am 2008;28(3):649–64.

8. Bloomberg GR, Chen E. The relationship of psychologic stress with childhood asthma. Immunol Allergy Clin North Am 2005;25(1):83–105.

9. Turyk ME, Hernandez E, Wright RJ, et al. Stressful life events and asthma in adolescents. Pediatr Allergy Immunol 2008;19(3):255–63.

10. Wright RJ, Steinbach SF. Violence: an unrecognized environmental exposure that may contribute to greater asthma morbidity in high risk inner-city populations [see comment]. Environ Health Perspect 2001;109(10):1085–9.

11. Sandberg S, Paton JY, Ahola S, et al. The role of acute and chronic stress in asthma attacks in children [see comment]. Lancet 2000;356(9234):982–7.

12. Lehrer P, Feldman J, Giardino N, et al. Psychological aspects of asthma. J Consult Clin Psychol 2002;70(3):691–711.

13. Mason JW. A historical view of the stress field. J Hum Stress 1975;1(2):22–36.

14. Holmes TH, Rahe RH. The social readjustment rating scale. J Psychosom Res 1967;11(2):213–8.

15. Cohen S, Kessler RC, Gordon LU. Measuring stress: a guide for health and social scientists. New York: Oxford University Press; 1995.

16. McGrath JE. Social and psychological factors in stress. Oxford: Holt, Rinehart, Winston; 1970.

17. Lazarus RS, Folkman S. Stress, appraisal, and coping. New York: Springer; 1984.

18. Lepore SJ, Cohen S, Kessler RC, et al. Measurement of chronic stressors. In: Cohen S, Kessler RC, Underwood Gordon L, editors. Measuring stress: a guide for health and social scientists. New York: Oxford University Press; 1997. p. 102–20.

19. Eckenrode J, Bolger N, Cohen S, et al. Daily and within-day event measurement. In: Cohen S, Kessler RC, Underwood Gordon L, editors. Measuring stress: a guide for health and social scientists. New York: Oxford University Press; 1997. p. 80–101.

20. Wright RJ, Rodriguez M, Cohen S. Review of psychosocial stress and asthma: an integrated biopsychosocial approach. Thorax 1998;53(12):1066–74.

21. Wright RJ, Cohen RT, Cohen S. The impact of stress on the development and expression of atopy. Curr Opin Allergy Clin Immunol 2005;5(1):23–9.

22. Kilpelainen M, Koskenvuo M, Helenius H, et al. Stressful life events promote the manifestation of asthma and atopic diseases. Clin Exp Allergy 2002;32(2):256–63.

23. Chen E, Fisher EB, Bacharier LB, et al. Socioeconomic status, stress, and immune markers in adolescents with asthma. Psychosom Med 2003;65(6):984–92.

24. DeMore M, Adams C, Wilson N, et al. Parenting stress, difficult child behavior, and use of routines in relation to adherence in pediatric asthma. Child Health Care 2005;34(4):245–59.
25. McQuaid EL, Fritz GK, Nassau JH, et al. Stress and airway resistance in children with asthma. J Psychosom Res 2000;49(4):239–45.
26. Smyth JM, Soefer MH, Hurewitz A, et al. Daily psychosocial factors predict levels and diurnal cycles of asthma symptomatology and peak flow. J Behav Med 1999; 22(2):179–93.
27. Chen E, Miller GE. Stress and inflammation in exacerbations of asthma. Brain Behav Immun 2007;21(8):993–9.
28. Salam MT, Islam T, Gilliland FD. Recent evidence for adverse effects of residential proximity to traffic sources on asthma. Curr Opin Pulm Med 2008;14(1):3–8.
29. Gordian ME, Haneuse S, Wakefield J. An investigation of the association between traffic exposure and the diagnosis of asthma in children. J Expo Sci Environ Epidemiol 2006;16(1):49–55.
30. Lin M, Chen Y, Villeneuve PJ, et al. Gaseous air pollutants and asthma hospitalization of children with low household income in Vancouver, British Columbia, Canada. Am J Epidemiol 2004;159(3):294–303.
31. O'Connor GT, Neas L, Vaughn B, et al. Acute respiratory health effects of air pollution on children with asthma in US inner cities. J Allergy Clin Immunol 2008;121(5):1133–9, e1131.
32. Rosenstreich DL, Eggleston P, Kattan M, et al. The role of cockroach allergy and exposure to cockroach allergen in causing morbidity among inner-city children with asthma [see comment]. N Engl J Med 1997;336(19):1356–63.
33. Barnes PJ. Th2 cytokines and asthma: an introduction. Respir Res 2001;2(2): 64–5.
34. Chung KF, Barnes PJ. Cytokines in asthma. Thorax 1999;54(9):825–57.
35. Chiou HH, Hsieh L-P. Parenting stress in parents of children with epilepsy and asthma. J Child Neurol 2008;23(3):301–6.
36. Busse WW, Lemanske RF Jr. Asthma. N Engl J Med 2001;344(5):350–62.
37. Chen E, Hanson MD, Paterson LQ, et al. Socioeconomic status and inflammatory processes in childhood asthma: the role of psychological stress. J Allergy Clin Immunol 2006;117(5):1014–20.
38. Miller GE, Gaudin A, Zysk E, et al. Parental support and cytokine activity in childhood asthma: the role of glucocorticoid sensitivity. J Allergy Clin Immunol 2009; 123(4):824–30.
39. Liu LY, Coe CL, Swenson CA, et al. School examinations enhance airway inflammation to antigen challenge. Am J Respir Crit Care Med 2002;165(8):1062–7.
40. Kang DH, Coe CL, Karaszewski J, et al. Relationship of social support to stress responses and immune function in healthy and asthmatic adolescents. Res Nurs Health 1998;21(2):117–28.
41. Miller BD, Wood BL. Psychophysiologic reactivity in asthmatic children: a cholinergically mediated confluence of pathways. J Am Acad Child Adolesc Psychiatry 1994;33(9):1236–45.
42. Rietveld S, Beest IV, Everaerd W. Stress-induced breathlessness in asthma. Psychol Med 1999;29(6):1359–66.
43. Chen E, Strunk RC, Bacharier LB, et al. Socioeconomic status associated with exhaled nitric oxide responses to acute stress in children with asthma. Brain Behav Immun 2010;24(3):444–50.
44. Shiffman S, Stone AA. Introduction to the special section: ecological momentary assessment in health psychology. Health Psychol 1998;17(1):3–5.

45. Turner RJ, Wheaton B, Cohen S, et al. Checklist measurement of stressful life events. In: Cohen S, Kessler RC, Underwood Gordon L, editors. Measuring stress: a guide for health and social scientists. New York: Oxford University Press; 1997. p. 29–58.

46. Cohen S, Kamarck T, Mermelstein R. A global measure of perceived stress. J Health Soc Behav 1983;24(4):385–96.

47. Wright RJ, Finn P, Contreras JP, et al. Chronic caregiver stress and IgE expression, allergen-induced proliferation, and cytokine profiles in a birth cohort predisposed to atopy. J Allergy Clin Immunol 2004;113(6):1051–7.

48. Chen E, Matthews KA. Development of the Cognitive Appraisal and Understanding of Social Events (CAUSE) videos. Health Psychol 2003;22(1):106–10.

49. Chen E, Miller GE, Walker HA, et al. Genome-wide transcriptional profiling linked to social class in asthma. Thorax 2009;64(1):38–43.

50. Rudolph KD, Hammen C. Age and gender as determinants of stress exposure, generation, and reactions in youngsters: a transactional perspective. Child Dev 1999;70(3):660–77.

51. Brown GW, Harris T. Social origins of depression: a study of psychiatric disorder in women. London: Tavistock Publications; 1978.

52. Hammen C. Generation of stress in the course of unipolar depression. J Abnorm Psychol 1991;100(4):555–61.

53. Wolf JM, Nicholls E, Chen E. Chronic stress, salivary cortisol, and alpha-amylase in children with asthma and healthy children. Biol Psychol 2008;78(1):20–8.

54. Chen E, Schreier HM, Strunk RC, et al. Chronic traffic-related air pollution and stress interact to predict biologic and clinical outcomes in asthma [see comment]. Environ Health Perspect 2008;116(7):970–5.

55. Sandberg S, Rutter M, Giles S, et al. Assessment of psychosocial experiences in childhood: methodological issues and some illustrative findings. J Child Psychol Psychiatry 1993;34(6):879–97.

56. Glen S, Simpson A, Drinnan D, et al. Testing the reliability of a new measure of life events and experiences in childhood: The Psychosocial Assessment of Childhood Experiences (PACE). Eur Child Adolesc Psychiatry 1993;2(2):98–110.

57. Sandberg S, Jarvenpaa S, Penttinen A, et al. Asthma exacerbations in children immediately following stressful life events: a Cox's hierarchical regression. Thorax 2004;59(12):1046–51 [Erratum appears in: Thorax 2005 Mar;60(3):261].

58. Shalowitz MU, Berry CA, Rasinski KA, et al. A new measure of contemporary life stress: development, validation, and reliability of the CRISYS. Health Serv Res 1998;33(5 Pt 1):1381–402.

59. Shalowitz MU, Berry CA, Quinn KA, et al. The relationship of life stressors and maternal depression to pediatric asthma morbidity in a subspecialty practice. Ambul Pediatr 2001;1(4):185–93.

60. Marin TJ, Chen E, Munch JA, et al. Double-exposure to acute stress and chronic family stress is associated with immune changes in children with asthma. Psychosom Med 2009;71(4):378–84.

61. Miller GE, Chen E. Life stress and diminished expression of genes encoding glucocorticoid receptor and beta2-adrenergic receptor in children with asthma. Proc Natl Acad Sci U S A 2006;103(14):5496–501.

62. Chen E, Chim LS, Strunk RC, et al. The role of the social environment in children and adolescents with asthma. Am J Respir Crit Care Med 2007;176(7):644–9.

Stress and Allergic Diseases

Ninabahen D. Dave, MBBS*, Lianbin Xiang, MD,
Kristina E. Rehm, PhD, Gailen D. Marshall Jr, MD, PhD

KEYWORDS

• Allergy • Asthma • Stress • Immunoregulation

Allergic diseases such as asthma, allergic rhinitis (AR), food allergies, and insect sting allergies have been described since early recorded history. A clinical condition with asthmalike symptoms was described 3500 years ago in an Egyptian manuscript dubbed the Ebers Papyrus.[1] In 1906, Austrian pediatrician Clemens von Pirquet first used the word *allergy* to describe the strange, non–disease-related symptoms that some diphtheria patients developed when treated with horse serum antitoxins.[2] Subsequently the field of clinical allergy developed, based on multiple discoveries: the clinical effectiveness of allergen immunotherapy,[3] mast cell granules as the major source of histamine in humans,[4] identification of IgE as the allergen-specific initiator of allergic reactions,[5] and the lipoxygenase-based leukotriene cascade as the clinically described slow-reacting substance of anaphylaxis.[6] These and other discoveries have led to the modern-day practice of allergy and clinical immunology, which cares for up to 30% of people in western societies who have various allergic diseases including hay fever (AR), asthma, atopic dermatitis, food allergy, drug allergy, and the life-threatening systemic mast cell–mediated reaction known as anaphylaxis.

Allergy has been defined as the result of immune reaction to specific types of mostly protein antigens known as allergens. Atopy, genetically mediated predisposition to produce specific IgE following exposure to allergens, is clinically defined as having evidence of allergic sensitization to at least 1 environmental allergen. Atopy is a fundamental component of the pathogenesis of allergic disorders. Although the clinical manifestations can be distinct between affected organs in a patient, and even the same organ among different patients, allergic diseases share a common pathophysiology resulting from immune dysregulation and subsequent potentially harmful inflammation (so-called hypersensitivity disease).

Supported in part by grants 1 CPI MP061018-02, 5 R21 AT002938-02 and 1 R21 HL96086-01 from the National Institutes of Health.
Laboratory of Behavioral Immunology Research, Division of Clinical Immunology and Allergy, Department of Medicine, The University of Mississippi Medical Center, 2500 North State Street, Jackson, MS 39216-4505, USA
* Corresponding author.
E-mail address: ndave@umc.edu

Immunol Allergy Clin N Am 31 (2011) 55–68
doi:10.1016/j.iac.2010.09.009
0889-8561/11/$ – see front matter © 2011 Elsevier Inc. All rights reserved.

immunology.theclinics.com

In recent decades, many studies have shown multiple links between nervous, endocrine, and immune systems.[7] Psychoneuroimmunology (PNI) has and continues to describe various links between behavior, neuroendocrine functions, immune responses, and health. Excessive psychological stress and allergic disorders have been linked in clinical practice for centuries. Many allergic conditions have long been considered to be psychosomatic disorders that had worse outcomes in patients with high levels of psychosocial stress. For example, asthma was commonly referred to in most early medical texts as asthma nervosa based on the belief that, in many children, it was the result of a conversion reaction from living with a histrionic mother.[8] Early descriptions of atopic dermatitis used the term neurodermatitis because of belief that the itch and scratch cycle that results in a rash was related primarily to nerves and emotion.

Thus, it is not surprising that allergy, one of the most prevalent of all human disease categories, and psychological stress are related. This article explores the relationships between allergic diseases and stress and suggests future mechanism-based research directions to develop therapeutic and even prophylactic approaches to disease management with stress-based interventions.

STRESS

Stress can be thought of as a psychophysiologic process that is a product of both the appraisal of a given situation to assess potential adversity and the ability (either perceived or actual) to cope with that potentially adverse situation.[8] The events/situations posing the potential threat are called stressors. Situations can be experiences in daily life, including daily hassles (ordinary stressors from interactions with family, neighborhood, school, or work place) as well as major life events, which may be either positive or negative such as a large promotion that requires significantly increased physical and mental effort or losing one's job resulting in financial crisis. Based on their duration, stressors are often considered acute (minutes to hours), subacute (less than 1 month duration), or chronic (months to years). Intensity of the stress, even when acute, may have longer-lasting effects that can overlap with a less intense stressor lasting for a longer period of time. Repetitive acute stressors (the same ones or even different ones) may, with time and intensity, have similar effects to that of a single long-term stressor.

PNI research focuses primarily on the understanding of the relationships between psychological stress perception (both conscious and subconscious) and downstream behavior, endocrine and immune changes occurring in response to that stress perception. The brain perceives and responds to stressors and determines both the behavioral and physiologic responses. The typical host response to isolated episodes of acute stress is adaptive for the protection of the host, whereas chronic stress can lead to dysregulation of the mediators and exacerbate underlying inflammatory disease pathophysiology. There are multiple reported factors that can affect this cause-and-effect relationship including genetic background (which may include gender and racial differences), previous life experiences, and past/present environmental exposures.[9] The same factors have been reported to have an effect on the incidence and severity of allergic diseases as well.

ADVERSE EFFECT OF STRESS ON HEALTH

A common clinical observation is the often adverse relationship between stress and human diseases.[10] Various sources have estimated that up to 75% of all visits to physician's offices are stress-related. This seems to be particularly true in relation to other immune-based dysfunctions such as increased susceptibility to infections and various autoimmune diseases. Stress is also implicated in morbidity and mortality of other inflammation-based diseases such as cancer, human immunodeficiency virus (HIV)/AIDS, inflammatory bowel disease, and even immune senescence associated with aging. Stress may also cause persistent increases in sympathetic nervous system activity, including increases in blood pressure, heart rate, and catecholamine secretion as well as platelet aggregation, which may explain, at least in part, the known association between stress, immune alteration, and cardiovascular disease. In addition, altered sleep can modulate the stress-health relationship. Sleep disturbance has been associated with adverse physical health outcomes including increased morbidity and mortality compared with the population with adequate pattern and duration of sleep. Other pathologies associated with allostatic overload from chronic stress include depression,[11] tendencies to unhealthy behavior,[12] diabetes,[13] dyslipidemia[13]; irritable bowel syndrome,[14] and cerebrovascular accidents.[15]

STRESS AND ALLERGIC DISEASE
Stress-induced Exacerbation of Existing Allergic Disease

Clinical observations implicating the adverse effects of psychological stress on disease activity in patients with allergy is supported by studies that have shown that allergic responses can be modulated by mood and psychological stressors. Gauci and colleagues[16] found a correlation between the Minnesota Multiphasic Personality Inventory distress-related scales and skin reactivity in response to allergen challenge. In addition, different studies have shown that the effect of life events, negative support, and current mood disorders were associated with increased rate of hospital admission for asthma,[17] and negative life events and negative ruminations were associated with asthma morbidity.[18] Behavior problems and family conflicts preceded the development of asthma in multiple pediatric populations.[19,20]

Another study showed enhancement of allergic inflammatory responses with natural stress exposure.[21] Sputum eosinophil levels in 20 otherwise healthy college students with asthma were evaluated before and after an allergen challenge. Although there were no baseline differences before antigen challenge at low (midsemester) and high (during final examinations) stress exposures, sputum eosinophil counts rose higher and persisted longer in response to allergen challenge during final examinations. In addition, blood eosinophil levels were significantly higher both before and after challenge during final examinations compared with the midsemester samples.

Stress and Incidence of Allergic Disease

The potential for adverse effects of maternal stress on immunity in a developing fetus and possible postnatal disease occurrence is concerning. Psychological maternal stress is increasingly considered a possible perinatal programming agent. Perinatal programming occurs when characteristics of the in utero environment, independent of genetic susceptibility, influence fetal development to permanently organize or imprint physiologic systems. Intrauterine stress hormone levels (both maternal and fetal) are believed to increase with prenatal maternal stress. Because fetal immunity initially is involved primarily in self-nonself programming to prevent future autoimmunity, such prenatal stress hormone exposure may alter natural immunoregulatory mechanisms such that the child has increased risk for developing various inflammatory diseases including allergy and asthma.

Various animal and human studies have shown a link between maternal stress and immune dysregulation in children. Wright and colleagues[22] reported that increased stress in early childhood was associated with an atopic immune profile in children predisposed to atopy-asthma (ie, positive family history for atopy). They have also shown that caregiver stress can increase the incidence of early childhood wheeze independent of caregiver smoking, breastfeeding behaviors, allergen exposure, birth weight, or lower respiratory tract infections.[22,23] These findings indicate a significant potential effect of psychological stress on childhood wheeze and subsequent development of clinical allergy and asthma. These studies and others support a strong role for stress in exacerbation and possible etiology of allergic diseases.

IMMUNOPATHOPHYSIOLOGY OF ALLERGIC DISEASE

IgE-mediated allergic disorders may manifest clinically as any combination of conjunctivitis, rhinitis, asthma, atopic dermatitis, food or drug intolerance, or anaphylaxis. It has been well recognized that atopic dermatitis and food allergies are often the earliest manifestation of atopic predisposition in a young child. Nearly 50% of children with atopic dermatitis develop asthma and 75% develop AR. The allergic march, a sequential or sometimes simultaneous expression of 2 or 3 of these allergic disorders in an individual, progresses from infancy to adolescence and adulthood.[24]

The prevalence of allergy and asthma has increased in nearly all countries worldwide and is more common in westernized and economically developed countries. As many as 1 in 3 individuals suffer from some form of allergic disorder.[25] Development of allergic disorders involves multiple factors including genetic components (family history), both indoor (dust mite, molds, animal danders) and outdoor (pollens, ozone, and diesel exhaust) environmental exposure, as well as other lifestyle factors including maternal diet, reproductive physiology and birth outcomes, breastfeeding, child nutrition and vitamin D level, obesity, physical activity, and psychological stress.

Atopic Dermatitis

Atopic dermatitis (AD) is a chronic relapsing inflammatory skin disease commonly associated with respiratory allergy.[26] It is the most common chronic skin disease of young children, with lifetime prevalence in US schoolchildren up to 17%. Itching and scratching are the hallmark of this disease. Itching is often worse at night leading to chronic sleep disturbance in the patient and immediate family members, and is a source of significant psychological and physiologic stress. When patients with AD become upset, they tend to itch even more, probably secondary to flushing of the skin as a result of vasodilatation induced by neurogenic peptides, followed by increased histamine and prostaglandin E2 release.[27] Distribution of the rash on the face and extensor aspects in infants and young children, changing to more flexural surface involvement in older ages is a classic finding of AD. About 95% of patients with AD become colonized by a ubiquitous pathogen, *Staphylococcus aureus*, which releases toxins that can act as superantigens and stimulate marked inflammatory responses as well as specific IgE production. Patients with AD are prone to recurrent bacterial (impetigo), fungal (tinea), and viral (herpes simplex molluscum contagiosum) skin infections. Allergens, irritants (wool, soap, detergents, heat, and humidity with sweating), infections, and certain foods can worsen eczema.[28,29] The effect on self-esteem and social interactions of both children and adults with this condition cannot be underestimated, and may account for some of the chronicity commonly seen in these patients.[30]

AR

AR is a debilitating disease that currently affects up to 30% of the world population. Classic symptoms of AR include profuse watery rhinorrhea, sneezing, itchy nose, and congestion. Postnasal drip might be present and cause cough or persistent throat clearing. Sometimes patients with AR can also experience itchy conjunctiva, ears, and throat. AR is generally classified as seasonal (SAR) and perennial (PAR), based on the presence or absence of seasonality and the source of allergens triggering the symptoms, but more recently has been classified based on duration and severity of symptoms as mild intermittent, mild persistent, moderate or severe intermittent, and moderate or severe persistent to aid with choice of therapy.

Nonallergic triggers such as strong odors, tobacco smoke, and temperature changes can stimulate symptoms in patients with AR similar to those induced by allergens., suggesting a hyperresponsiveness that is more commonly reported in lower airways. Neural reflex arcs in the upper airways, when challenged with allergens, can incite lower airway bronchospasm. These observations led to the concept of one linked airway, which addresses the observed connection between nasal and pulmonary symptoms in allergic individuals.[31] Patients with AR can often have sleep impairment because of nasal obstruction, which typically worsens at night. Fatigue, malaise, and impairment of work and school performance are common when AR symptoms are severe.[32] Patients with AR are more prone to upper respiratory infections during periods of high psychological stress.[33]

Asthma

Asthma is defined as a chronic inflammatory disorder of the airways in which many cells and cellular elements play a role. The chronic inflammation causes an associated increase in airway hyperresponsiveness that leads to recurrent episodes of wheezing, breathlessness, chest tightness, and coughing, particularly at night or in the early morning. These episodes are usually associated with widespread but variable airflow obstruction that is often reversible either spontaneously or with treatment.[34] Based on results from NHIS 2005, an estimated 32.6 million Americans have received an asthma diagnosis during their lifetime, an increase in prevalence of 16% from 1997.[35] Atopy, particularly to house dust mites and cockroaches, and a family history of allergy or asthma are known risk factors for asthma. Common symptoms described by patients include cough, wheezing, chest tightness, dyspnea, and occasionally chest pain. In up to 15% of patients with asthma, a dry cough may be the only presenting respiratory symptom. Exercise-induced bronchospasm is present in almost 90% of all asthmatics resulting from rapid change of airway temperatures with increased tidal volumes and mouth breathing. Any and all of these symptoms have been reported to be worsened in patients with asthma experiencing high stress levels.

Acute exacerbation of asthma can be triggered by upper and lower respiratory tract infections (specially viruses such as rhinovirus, influenza, parainfluenza, respiratory syncitial viruses), changes in the weather, significant allergen exposure in sensitized individuals, cold air, exercise, various stressful situations, and hormonal changes related to menses in some women. Approximately 5000 deaths from asthma occur annually in the United States.

ALTERED IMMUNITY IN ALLERGIC DISEASES

For the purposes of this discussion, allergy or immediate hypersensitivity describes a series of immune-based reactions occurring as a result of the induction of allergen-specific IgE, which binds to mast cells via high affinity FcεR1 receptors. Subsequent reexposure to the inciting allergen causes a cross-linking of the mast cell–bound IgE with activation and release of the mast cell contents such as histamine, leukotrines, tryptase, chymase, kininogenase, and heparin within 5 to 60 minutes of exposure. These mediators can induce vasodilatation and vascular leaks, causing mucosal edema, increased mucus gland secretions, nasal and/or bronchial congestion, and occlusion resulting in various clinical signs and symptoms. Late phase allergic reactions can occur 6 to 24 hours after initial exposure following the recruitment and migration of inflammatory cells such as eosinophils, basophils, neutrophils, T lymphocytes, and macrophages to the target tissues (skin, nose, lung, gastrointestinal tract, and/or blood vessels). These result in more persistent symptoms. Th2 cytokines play a critical role in orchestrating ongoing inflammation.

Chronic changes seen in the airways of asthmatics include smooth muscle hypertrophy and hyperplasia, goblet cell hyperplasia, submucosal gland hypertrophy, neovascularization, thickening of reticular basement membrane, and fibrotic changes with collagen deposition.[36] Airway smooth muscle hyperresponsiveness is another hallmark of asthma that might precede, accompany, and sometimes be independent of airway inflammation, suggesting heterogeneity of asthma phenotypes. Increased transepithelial water losses, defective skin barrier function, allergen- and infection-induced inflammation, and abnormal regeneration of damaged skin are the characteristics of AD.[29]

As already discussed, the production of the IgE is under the direct control of type 2 cytokine production with IL-4 and IL-13 being responsible for the isotype switch from IgM to IgE. IL-4 is also a mast cell growth factor and IL-5 is a major chemotactic, growth and activation factor for eosinophils, which are a central component of allergic inflammation.[37] Thus, clinical allergic diseases can be viewed as immunoregulatory imbalances in which Th2 cytokines predominate.[38]

Dysregulation of Th1 and Th2 cytokine balance plays a central role in the immunopathology of allergic diseases. Allergen-specific T-cell clones from atopic patients have a much higher percentage of Th2 or Th0 type compared with healthy individuals, who tend to have more Th1.[39,40] Treatment of AR with allergen immunotherapy has been shown to result in a shift in the overall Th1 and Th2 cytokine levels toward a more balanced Th1/Th2 response, which correlates with decreases in clinical disease activity.[41] These mechanism studies support the theory that physiologic states associated with the type II cytokine environment could exacerbate asthmatic and allergic diseases.

Chronic psychosocial stress has been shown to be associated with an altered Th1/Th2 balance toward a Th2 predominance, therefore it is not surprising from an immune standpoint that stress can exacerbate allergic diseases such as AR, AD, and asthma. Such observations led to interventions for these diseases based on the notion of managing (if not reducing) stress as a means to control symptoms and, perhaps in the future, preventing the appearance of allergic diseases in the most susceptible individuals (**Fig. 1**).

MANAGEMENT OF ALLERGIC DISEASE

Clinical principles for managing allergic diseases include

1. Avoidance of exposure to known allergic and nonallergic triggers
2. Controlled exposure to allergens that cannot be totally avoided (ie, airborne pollens, mold spores, dust mite proteins)
3. Pharmacotherapy to treat mast cell–mediated symptoms and reduce allergic inflammation
4. Allergen immunotherapy for upper and lower airway disease in selected individuals.

Identification of allergens to which an individual is sensitive is typically accomplished by in vitro (ImmunoCAP-RAST) or in vivo (skin prick or intradermal skin testing)

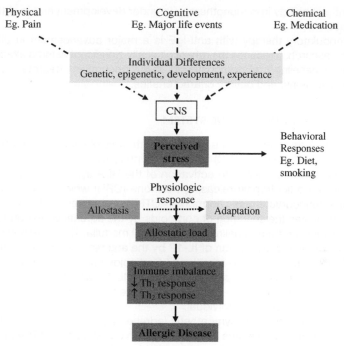

Fig. 1. Stress-allergic disease paradigm.

assays when feasible, which is then correlated with the clinical history of symptoms. Environmental control can improve the symptoms of susceptible patients with allergic diseases.[42] The general goal of pharmacotherapy for any disease is to minimize the effect of the disease on the patient's life with minimal adverse side effects of the medications. There are many different types of medications used to treat allergy and asthma but corticosteroids are the most effective antiinflammatory medications. Corticosteroids exert their antiinflammatory effects by suppressing the expression of a host of inflammatory mediators (growth factors, cytokines, chemokines) and inflammatory enzymes involved in the metabolism of arachidonic acid and nitric oxide. Topical forms of corticosteroids (ie, inhaled steroids for asthma, intranasal steroid sprays for AR, and topical steroid creams and ointments for allergic dermatitis) represent first-line therapy in the everyday management of allergic diseases. In addition, short courses of systemic corticosteroids are typically used for acute exacerbations of allergic diseases. Inhaled bronchodilators (β2-agonist) and anticholinergics are also used in the management of acute asthma exacerbations. Antihistamines in oral, intranasal, and ocular forms as well as leukotriene receptor antagonists are also used in the management of various allergic diseases.

Immunotherapy for inhaled allergens induces regulatory T cells that dampen the allergic responses to allergens. Two forms of immunotherapy, subcutaneous immunotherapy (SCIT) and sublingual immunotherapy (SLIT), are in use currently. SCIT, the conventional immunotherapy, involves injecting gradually increasing doses of an allergen to which a given patient is sensitive and has a history of problems on exposure, followed by maintenance therapy with the same allergen. Studies showed that the global assessment of improvement with SLIT was significantly better than placebo although only half the difference was recorded in the SCIT study.[43,44] Use of recombinant technology in immunotherapy is under development and is at the experimental phase.

Immunomodulatory therapy with anti-IgE is a major advancement in allergy and immunology research. It reduces the rate of clinically significant asthma exacerbations irrespective of baseline oral corticosteroid use, concomitant treatment with other controller medications, and patient characteristics.

EFFECT OF STRESS ON THE IMMUNE SYSTEM

The link between the brain and the immune system involves 2 main pathways: the autonomic nervous system (ANS) and the hyphophyseal-pituitary-adrenal (HPA) axis. Perception of stress leads to activation of the HPA system, which begins with the secretion of corticotrophin-releasing hormone (CRH) which in turn induces the secretion of adrenocorticotrophic hormone (ACTH) by the anterior lobe of the pituitary lobe. ACTH activates the secretion of corticoids by the adrenal cortex and catecholamines (adrenalin and noradrenalin) by the adrenal medulla. The catecholamines and corticoids suppress the production of IL-12 by the antigen-presenting cells, which is a primary Th1 cytokine-inducing stimulus.[45] Corticoids can also exert a direct effect on Th2 cells thus increasing the production of IL-4, IL-10, and IL-13.[46] The end result is the predominance of a Th2 cell–mediated response that favors an allergic inflammatory response in a susceptible individual.

The ANS is composed of the sympathetic (adrenergic, noradrenergic) and the parasympathetic (cholinergic) systems in the central nervous system (CNS) with noradrenalin and acetyl choline as neurotransmitters, respectively, and the nonadrenergic, noncholinergic (peptidergic) system primarily located in the gastrointestinal tract. The main peptides of this system are vasoactive intestinal peptides (VIP), substance P (SP), and calcitonin gene-related peptide (CGRP). The innervation of important organs and systems related to the immune system such as the liver, spleen, thymus gland, bone marrow, lymph nodes, skin, digestive tract, and respiratory apparatus is by postsynaptic ANS.[47] Most immune system cells have surface membrane receptors for varying combinations of neurotransmitters, neuropeptides, and hormones.[48]

The CNS modulates the immune system through neurotransmitters (acetyl choline, noradrenalin, serotonin, histamine, γ-aminobutyric acid, glutamic acid), neuropeptides (ACTH, prolactin, vasopressin, bradykinin, somatostatin, VIP, SP, neuropeptide Y, encephalin, endorphin), neurologic growth factors (neuron growth factor), and hormones (adrenalin and corticoids), whereas the immune system can also modulate CNS function via various molecules including cytokines (tumor necrosis factor alpha [TNFα] and beta [TGFβ]), chemokines (interferons) and nitric oxide.[49] Perception of acute stress stimulates the locus ceruleus, which secretes noradrenalin. Noradrenalin activates the sympathetic nervous system leading to decreased production of IL-12 as described earlier.

Neuropeptides including SP, CGRP, and VIP are potent vasodilators and also increase vascular permeability. SP increases the production of TNFα and IL-12 by monocytes and macrophages. SP and CRH can degranulate mast cells within inflammatory foci. All of these processes lead to inflammatory changes.[50]

SP and CGRP have been identified in bronchial mucosa as neurogenic inflammatory agents.[51] In addition, neurokinin-1, a receptor for SP, is located on bronchial vessels, bronchial smooth muscle, epithelial cells, submucosal glands, and immune cells. Stress likely exerts its effect on the bronchial mucosa of asthmatics by varying combinations of effects on the number and function of various immune/inflammatory cells, as well as direct action on the bronchial mucosa.[52]

Increased tissue levels of neurotrophins, acting as nerve growth factors, have been described in different respiratory and dermatologic allergic disorders. They act on immune cells, structural cells (keratinocytes, epithelial cells) and can increase angiogenesis.[53] Eosinophils and the submucosal glands of the nasal mucosa are a major source of neurotrophins,[54] which have been shown to regulate eosinophil survival in the lungs, increase production of specific IgE, and change the cytokine profile toward Th2 predominance.

These findings and others demonstrate that interactions between the CNS and immune systems are complex and bidirectional.

ADDRESSING STRESS IN COMPREHENSIVE ALLERGIC DISEASE MANAGEMENT

Similar to allergic diseases, progression of the other immune-based diseases such as cardiovascular disease, diabetes mellitus, development of AIDS in HIV-positive patients and certain malignancies has been suggested for high-stress populations. Thus, it follows that managing stress in these patients could be expected to have salutatory effects on their underlying disease course.

Strategies for stress management as part of a comprehensive treatment plan should involve identification of the high-risk population or, ideally, individuals. Current efforts are underway in our group and others to identify biomarkers that would categorize individuals into risk categories for adverse effects of psychological stress on their immune system, which, in turn, would affect the risk for or activity of underlying immune-based diseases. The categorization would be followed by (ideally) individualized prophylactic interventions in the highest at-risk individuals to prevent immune-based diseases or therapeutic intervention in individuals with disease with the intent of minimizing the immunoregulatory imbalance that characterizes chronic stress-induced immune changes.

Stress reduction/elimination would be the most desirable intervention but is often difficult to achieve in our fast-paced high-pressure societies. Methods (psychological, physiologic, pharmacologic, or some combination) to improve individual coping abilities to stressful situations are more likely to be clinically valuable as the core of interventional strategies for stress management.[55]

Many studies have shown the encouraging effects of psychological interventions on clinical outcome in allergic diseases. Smyth and colleagues[56] showed that expressive writing about stressful events was associated with symptom reduction in patients with asthma. Biofeedback as well as mental imagery has a positive role in asthma management.[57–59] In a systematic review, Huntley and colleagues[60] described that relaxation therapy had a positive effect on asthma outcomes. Psychotherapy can reduce the number of asthma exacerbations and emergency visits in patients with depression and asthma.[61] Although evidence suggests that these interventions restore a more normal Th1/Th2 balance, further research is warranted to prove a direct link between clinical improvement and immune changes after psychological interventions in allergic diseases.

Physiologic interventions for allergic diseases include various forms of exercise programs as well as complementary and alternative medicine techniques such as acupuncture, chiropractic, and applied kinesiology, all of which may work, at least in part, by their effect on the underlying stress of the individual. So far, well-designed studies have not shown a clear benefit of complementary and alternative medicine interventions, perhaps secondary to the robust placebo effect with a subsequent psychophysiologic effect on immunity[62,63] and thus likely on allergic diseases.[64] Based on the severity of the underlying dysfunction, exercise had varied effects on immune function. Exercise training programs are well tolerated in children with mild-to-moderate asthma and improve both aerobic and anaerobic fitness.[65] Exercise rehabilitation programs improve aerobic conditioning and ventilatory capacity, and decrease the hyperpnea of exercise that occurs in patients with mild asthma.[66] However, as a caution, excessive exercise can lead to an exacerbation of disease in patients with poorly controlled asthma.

Reported pharmacologic interventions for stress have mainly included psychoactive agents. Both tricyclic and selective serotonin reuptake inhibitor antidepressants may have a therapeutic role in asthma by suppressing production of proinflammatory cytokines, inducing production of antiinflammatory molecules and/or preventing the effects of these inflammatory molecules on the brain.[67] Both adult and child/adolescent populations with asthma seem to have a high prevalence of anxiety disorders.[68] In addition, anxiolytic drugs may be beneficial in increasing the quality of asthma therapy in asthmatics with anxiety disorder.[69]

Psychological stress increases superoxide release.[70] This finding suggests a potential prophylactic role of antioxidant agents such as vitamins C and E against stress-induced immune changes. Studies have shown vitamin C and vitamin E can reduce immunoregulatory imbalances noted in stressed individuals.[71]

Thus, many different approaches with proven or likely beneficial effects are available to modulate stress and thus immune function and have positive effects in patients with allergy.

FUTURE DIRECTIONS

Although the adverse role of psychological stress in allergic disease activity has long been suspected by clinicians, recent research has found more direct mechanistic links between stress and immunity. Future research should include development of ways to identify high-risk individuals as well as more accurate assessment of the specific effect of stress on various regulatory and effector components of the immune system and resulting allergic diseases.

CONCLUDING REMARKS

From the available evidence, it seems apparent that chronic stress in susceptible individuals can favor the manifestation of allergic disease and exacerbate as well as complicate the control of existing allergic diseases. Current research has delivered anatomic as well as physiologic evidence of intense communication between neuroendocrine mediators, nerve fibers, and immune cells in allergic diseases. There is a bidirectional relationship between psychosocial factors and allergic disorders. This suggests that optimal management of allergic disorders must involve a multipronged approach including psychological interventions as well as conventional physical and pharmacologic therapies.

REFERENCES

1. Ebers G. Das hermetische buch uber die arzneimittel der slten aegypter. Leipzig (Germany): Henrichs; 1875 [in German].
2. Bukantz SC. Clemens von Pirquet and the concept of allergie. J Allergy Clin Immunol 2002;109(4):724–6.
3. Noon L. Prophylactic inoculation against hay fever. Int Arch Allergy Appl Immunol 1953;4(4):285–8.
4. Riley JF, West GB. The presence of histamine in tissue mast cells. J Physiol 1953; 120(4):528–37.

5. Kirkpatrick CH. The Ishizakas and the search for reaginic antibodies. J Allergy Clin Immunol 2005;115(3):642–4.
6. Dahlen SE, Hedqvist P, Hammarstrom S, et al. Leukotrienes are potent constrictors of human bronchi. Nature 1980;288(5790):484–6.
7. Marshall GD. Neuroendocrine mechanisms of immune dysregulation: applications to allergy and asthma. Ann Allergy Asthma Immunol 2004;93(2 Suppl 1):S11–7.
8. Osler W. The principles and practice of medicine. Edinburgh (UK): YJ Pentland; 1892.
9. McEwen BS. Central effects of stress hormones in health and disease: understanding the protective and damaging effects of stress and stress mediators. Eur J Pharmacol 2008;583(2–3):174–85.
10. McEwen BS, Stellar E. Stress and the individual. Mechanisms leading to disease. Arch Intern Med 1993;153(18):2093–101.
11. Clays E, De Bacquer D, Leynen F, et al. Job stress and depression symptoms in middle-aged workers–prospective results from the Belstress study. Scand J Work Environ Health 2007;33(4):252–9.
12. Muller N, Ackenheil M. Psychoneuroimmunology and the cytokine action in the CNS: implications for psychiatric disorders. Prog Neuropsychopharmacol Biol Psychiatry 1998;22(1):1–33.
13. Golden SH. A review of the evidence for a neuroendocrine link between stress, depression and diabetes mellitus. Curr Diabetes Rev 2007;3(4):252–9.
14. Blanchard EB, Lackner JM, Jaccard J, et al. The role of stress in symptom exacerbation among IBS patients. J Psychosom Res 2008;64(2):119–28.
15. Harmsen P, Lappas G, Rosengren A, et al. Long-term risk factors for stroke: twenty-eight years of follow-up of 7457 middle-aged men in Goteborg, Sweden. Stroke 2006;37(7):1663–7.
16. Gauci M, King MG, Saxarra H, et al. A Minnesota Multiphasic Personality Inventory profile of women with allergic rhinitis. Psychosom Med 1993;55(6):533–40.
17. Wainwright NW, Surtees PG, Wareham NJ, et al. Psychosocial factors and incident asthma hospital admissions in the EPIC-Norfolk cohort study. Allergy 2007;62(5):554–60.
18. Wright RJ. Alternative modalities for asthma that reduce stress and modify mood states: evidence for underlying psychobiologic mechanisms. Ann Allergy Asthma Immunol 2004;93(2 Suppl 1):S18–23.
19. Calam R, Gregg L, Simpson A, et al. Behavior problems antecede the development of wheeze in childhood: a birth cohort study. Am J Respir Crit Care Med 2005;171(4):323–7.
20. Stevenson J. Relationship between behavior and asthma in children with atopic dermatitis. Psychosom Med 2003;65(6):971–5.
21. Liu LY, Coe CL, Swenson CA, et al. School examinations enhance airway inflammation to antigen challenge. Am J Respir Crit Care Med 2002;165(8):1062–7.
22. Wright RJ, Finn P, Contreras JP, et al. Chronic caregiver stress and IgE expression, allergen-induced proliferation, and cytokine profiles in a birth cohort predisposed to atopy. J Allergy Clin Immunol 2004;113(6):1051–7.
23. Wright RJ, Cohen S, Carey V, et al. Parental stress as a predictor of wheezing in infancy: a prospective birth-cohort study. Am J Respir Crit Care Med 2002;165(3):358–65.
24. Hahn EL, Bacharier LB. The atopic march: the pattern of allergic disease development in childhood. Immunol Allergy Clin North Am 2005;25(2):231–46, v.
25. Peroni DG, Piacentini GL, Alfonsi L, et al. Rhinitis in pre-school children: prevalence, association with allergic diseases and risk factors. Clin Exp Allergy 2003;33(10):1349–54.

26. Leung DY, Boguniewicz M, Howell MD, et al. New insights into atopic dermatitis. J Clin Invest 2004;113(5):651–7.
27. Ostlere LS, Cowen T, Rustin MH. Neuropeptides in the skin of patients with atopic dermatitis. Clin Exp Dermatol 1995;20(6):462–7.
28. Leung DY, Bieber T. Atopic dermatitis. Lancet 2003;361(9352):151–60.
29. Leung DY, Jain N, Leo HL. New concepts in the pathogenesis of atopic dermatitis. Curr Opin Immunol 2003;15(6):634–8.
30. Lapidus CS, Kerr PE. Social impact of atopic dermatitis. Med Health R I 2001; 84(9):294–5.
31. Blaiss MS. Rhinitis-asthma connection: epidemiologic and pathophysiologic basis. Allergy Asthma Proc 2005;26(1):35–40.
32. Meltzer EO. Quality of life in adults and children with allergic rhinitis. J Allergy Clin Immunol 2001;108(Suppl 1):S45–53.
33. Jaber R. Respiratory and allergic diseases: from upper respiratory tract infections to asthma. Prim Care 2002;29(2):231–61.
34. National Institutes of Health (NIH) NHL. Global initiative for asthma. Global strategy for asthma management and prevention. Bethesda (MD): NIH; 2002.
35. NHIS. National Health Interview Survey (NHIS 2005). Hyattsville (MD): National Center for Health Statistics (NCHS), Centers for Disease Control and Prevention; 2005.
36. James A. Airway remodeling in asthma. Curr Opin Pulm Med 2005;11(1):1–6.
37. Weltman JK, Karim AS. IL-5: biology and potential therapeutic applications. Expert Opin Investig Drugs 2000;9(3):491–6.
38. Ngoc PL, Gold DR, Tzianabos AO, et al. Cytokines, allergy, and asthma. Curr Opin Allergy Clin Immunol 2005;5(2):161–6.
39. Romagnani S. T-cell subsets (Th1 versus Th2). Ann Allergy Asthma Immunol 2000;85(1):9–18 [quiz: 18, 21].
40. Romagnani S, Maggi E, Parronchi P, et al. Increased numbers of Th2-like CD4+ T cells in target organs and in the allergen-specific repertoire of allergic patients. Possible role of IL-4 produced by non-T cells. Int Arch Allergy Appl Immunol 1991;94(1–4):133–6.
41. Schmidt-Weber CB, Blaser K. Immunological mechanisms in specific immunotherapy. Springer Semin Immunopathol 2004;25(3–4):377–90.
42. Simpson A, John SL, Jury F, et al. Endotoxin exposure, CD14, and allergic disease: an interaction between genes and the environment. Am J Respir Crit Care Med 2006;174(4):386–92.
43. Khinchi MS, Poulsen LK, Carat F, et al. Clinical efficacy of sublingual and subcutaneous birch pollen allergen-specific immunotherapy: a randomized, placebo-controlled, double-blind, double-dummy study. Allergy 2004;59(1):45–53.
44. Lima MT, Wilson D, Pitkin L, et al. Grass pollen sublingual immunotherapy for seasonal rhinoconjunctivitis: a randomized controlled trial. Clin Exp Allergy 2002;32(4):507–14.
45. Elenkov IJ, Chrousos GP. Stress hormones, Th1/Th2 patterns, pro/anti-inflammatory cytokines and susceptibility to disease. Trends Endocrinol Metab 1999;10(9): 359–68.
46. DeKruyff RH, Fang Y, Umetsu DT. Corticosteroids enhance the capacity of macrophages to induce Th2 cytokine synthesis in CD4+ lymphocytes by inhibiting IL-12 production. J Immunol 1998;160(5):2231–7.
47. Felten SY, Felten DL, Bellinger DL, et al. Noradrenergic sympathetic innervation of lymphoid organs. Prog Allergy 1988;43:14–36.

48. Steinman L. Elaborate interactions between the immune and nervous systems. Nat Immunol 2004;5(6):575–81.

49. Mix E, Goertsches R, Zettl UK. Immunology and neurology. J Neurol 2007;254 (Suppl 2):II2–7.

50. Elenkov IJ. Neurohormonal-cytokine interactions: implications for inflammation, common human diseases and well-being. Neurochem Int 2008;52(1–2):40–51.

51. Lamb JP, Sparrow MP. Three-dimensional mapping of sensory innervation with substance p in porcine bronchial mucosa: comparison with human airways. Am J Respir Crit Care Med 2002;166(9):1269–81.

52. Joachim RA, Sagach V, Quarcoo D, et al. Neurokinin-1 receptor mediates stress-exacerbated allergic airway inflammation and airway hyperresponsiveness in mice. Psychosom Med 2004;66(4):564–71.

53. Nockher WA, Renz H. Neurotrophins in allergic diseases: from neuronal growth factors to intercellular signaling molecules. J Allergy Clin Immunol 2006;117(3):583–9.

54. Wu X, Myers AC, Goldstone AC, et al. Localization of nerve growth factor and its receptors in the human nasal mucosa. J Allergy Clin Immunol 2006;118(2):428–33.

55. Barton C, Clarke D, Sulaiman N, et al. Coping as a mediator of psychosocial impediments to optimal management and control of asthma. Respir Med 2003; 97(7):747–61.

56. Smyth J, Helm R. Focused expressive writing as self-help for stress and trauma. J Clin Psychol 2003;59(2):227–35.

57. Lehrer PM, Vaschillo E, Vaschillo B, et al. Biofeedback treatment for asthma. Chest 2004;126(2):352–61.

58. Epstein GN, Halper JP, Barrett EA, et al. A pilot study of mind-body changes in adults with asthma who practice mental imagery. Altern Ther Health Med 2004; 10(4):66–71.

59. Freeman LW, Welton D. Effects of imagery, critical thinking, and asthma education on symptoms and mood state in adult asthma patients: a pilot study. J Altern Complement Med 2005;11(1):57–68.

60. Huntley A, White AR, Ernst E. Relaxation therapies for asthma: a systematic review. Thorax 2002;57(2):127–31.

61. Lehrer P, Feldman J, Giardino N, et al. Psychological aspects of asthma. J Consult Clin Psychol 2002;70(3):691–711.

62. Jamison JR. Psychoneuroendoimmunology: the biological basis of the placebo phenomenon? J Manipulative Physiol Ther 1996;19(7):484–7.

63. Rossi EL. Psychosocial genomics: gene expression, neurogenesis, and human experience in mind-body medicine. Adv Mind Body Med 2002;18(2):22–30.

64. Markham AW, Wilkinson JM. Complementary and alternative medicines (CAM) in the management of asthma: an examination of the evidence. J Asthma 2004; 41(2):131–9.

65. Counil FP, Varray A, Matecki S, et al. Training of aerobic and anaerobic fitness in children with asthma. J Pediatr 2003;142(2):179–84.

66. Hallstrand TS, Bates PW, Schoene RB. Aerobic conditioning in mild asthma decreases the hyperpnea of exercise and improves exercise and ventilatory capacity. Chest 2000;118(5):1460–9.

67. Krommydas G, Gourgoulianis KI, Karamitsos K, et al. Therapeutic value of anti-depressants in asthma. Med Hypotheses 2005;64(5):938–40.

68. Katon WJ, Richardson L, Lozano P, et al. The relationship of asthma and anxiety disorders. Psychosom Med 2004;66(3):349–55.

69. Haida M, Itoh K. [Clinical effect of alprazolam and trazodone on bronchial asthmatics with anxiety disorder]. Arerugi 1997;46(10):1058–71 [in Japanese].

70. Kang DH, McCarthy DO. The effect of psychological stress on neutrophil superoxide release. Res Nurs Health 1994;17(5):363–70.

71. Wakikawa A, Utsuyama M, Wakabayashi A, et al. Vitamin E enhances the immune functions of young but not old mice under restraint stress. Exp Gerontol 1999; 34(7):853–62.

Stressor-Induced Alterations of Adaptive Immunity to Vaccination and Viral Pathogens

Nicole D. Powell, PhD[a,b], Rebecca G. Allen, BS[a,b,c],
Amy R. Hufnagle, BS[a,b], John F. Sheridan, PhD[a,b,c],
Michael T. Bailey, PhD[a,b],*

KEYWORDS

- Psychoneuroimmunology • Stress • Influenza vaccine
- Antibody response

Scientists and physicians who are asked about significant achievements in public health often rank the development of vaccines at the top of the list. In fact, the Centers for Disease Control have listed vaccination as one of the 10 greatest health achievements in recorded history.[1] This fact is not surprising, given that once devastating diseases, such as polio, rubella, and smallpox (to name a few) have been largely contained or eliminated. Protective immunity, however, does not always develop on vaccination, and it is now known that genetic, environmental, and psychosocial factors can influence the development of protective immunity. The purpose of this review is to describe basic mechanisms involved in vaccination, to describe clinical studies linking psychosocial stressor to protective immunity induced by vaccines, and finally to describe animal studies that have attempted to define mechanisms linking the stress response to alterations in adaptive immunity.

VACCINES

Active vaccination is the process in which immunogenic material from a pathogenic microbe is administered to individuals to induce protective immunity against a disease. The first documented use of vaccination occurred in the late 1700s when Edward

---

[a] Division of Oral Biology, College of Dentistry, The Ohio State University, Columbus, OH 43210, USA
[b] Institute for Behavioral Medicine Research, College of Medicine, The Ohio State University, 257 IBMR Building, 460 Medical Center Drive, Columbus, OH 43210, USA
[c] Integrated Biomedical Sciences Graduate Program, College of Medicine, The Ohio State University, Columbus, OH 43210, USA
* Corresponding author. Institute for Behavioral Medicine Research, The Ohio State University, 257 IBMR Building, 460 Medical Center Drive, Columbus, OH 43210.
E-mail address: Michael.bailey@osumc.edu

Immunol Allergy Clin N Am 31 (2011) 69–79
doi:10.1016/j.iac.2010.09.002
0889-8561/11/$ – see front matter © 2011 Elsevier Inc. All rights reserved.

Jenner observed that resistance to smallpox could be induced by exposure to cowpox. To prove this concept, Jenner administered the pus from a cowpox lesion to an 8-year-old boy. Six weeks later, Jenner inoculated the boy's arm with smallpox, and as expected, the young boy did not develop any symptoms of the smallpox.[2] This seminal observation helped trigger the development of immunology, and was the first evidence that protective immunity could be induced through vaccinations.[2]

Over the next century, vaccines were developed to protect against other devastating diseases (most notably rabies vaccines by Louis Pasteur), triggering a quest to determine the scientific basis of vaccination. It is now recognized that vaccines work by inducing the development of adaptive immunity (both cellular and humoral components) to the microbe being vaccinated against. Although immunity to the cowpox virus was sufficiently similar to the smallpox (ie, variola) virus to elicit protective immunity without inducing any symptoms of either the cowpox or the smallpox, this is by no means the norm. Thus, the challenge for vaccine development and effective immunization is to develop a vaccine that has the necessary immunogenic potential to stimulate a robust adaptive immune response and yet does not cause disease.

Vaccine Types

At present, there are 3 strategies for vaccine preparation that elicit the desired immune response.[2] Live attenuated vaccines are composed of intact microbes that have been attenuated by treating the viruses in a way that reduces their virulence disease while maintaining immunogenicity. Examples of live attenuated vaccines include measles/mumps/rubella (MMR), nasally administered influenza vaccine, and oral polio vaccine. This type of vaccine is advantageous because it causes a mild, often asymptomatic infection that stimulates both innate and adaptive immune responses, leading to significant antiviral protection. Some microbes, however, easily revert to their virulent form from this induced attenuated form. Thus, only microbes with low reversion rates can be used as live attenuated vaccines.

If attenuation is not possible, an alternative form of the microbe that will still induce a strong immune response is a killed or inactivated microbe vaccine. In this case, the microbe is killed or inactivated so that it cannot replicate and cause disease. The microbe can either be left intact (eg, whole virus vaccines) or can be dissociated, such as with a detergent (eg, split-virus vaccines). Split-virus vaccines contain all of the dissociated viral particles. The most commonly used killed vaccine is the influenza vaccine, which is a split-virus trivalent vaccine comprised of viral components from 3 different types of influenza virus. While safer than live, attenuated vaccines, the immune response to killed vaccines is often effective for shorter periods of time and induces more limited protection.

A third vaccine form is the subunit vaccine. Subunit vaccines contain only the portions of the pathogen that the immune system recognizes and reacts to. For example, immune system recognition of the capsular antigens of *Neisseria meningitides* results in protective immunity.[3] Thus, meningococcal vaccines are subunit vaccines that contain *N meningitides* capsular antigens.[3] Other commonly used capsular vaccines include the DTaP vaccine to protect against diphtheria, tetanus, and pertussis, as well as the pneumococcal vaccines to protect against *Streptococcus pneumoniae*, the *Haemophilus influenzae* type B vaccine (Hib), and vaccines against hepatitis A and B. Although this type of vaccine eliminates all safety concerns and is easily stored and stable for long periods of time, subunit and conjugate vaccines do not often induce the development of antigen-specific T lymphocytes.[4] As a result, cell-mediated immunity is not strongly activated.

Vaccine-Induced Immunization

Protective immunity involves the effective development of adaptive immunity. While neutralizing antibodies produced by B cells are commonly viewed as the crucial component of protective immunity, T-cell responses are also essential.[4] Because many studies assessing the impact of psychosocial factors on the immune response to vaccines have involved influenza vaccination, the immune response to influenza and the influenza vaccine is outlined here. It should be noted, however, that the immune response is similar to other types of inactivated vaccines.

Respiratory epithelial cells are the primary target for influenza virus.[5,6] On infection, these cells produce chemokines and cytokines to recruit and activate cells of the innate immune system. The innate immune cells, primarily macrophages and dendritic cells (DCs), are then responsible for initiating the adaptive immune response. This response occurs when the macrophages and DCs phagocytose and degrade the virus so that viral antigen can be expressed along with major histocompatibility complex class I (MHCI) or MHCII. The macrophages and DCs migrate to draining lymph nodes where they come into contact with T cells. Viral antigen presentation in the context of MHC, along with recognition of costimulatory cues, causes virus-specific CD4+ and CD8+ T cells to clonally expand in the lymph nodes. These antigen-specific T cells can then leave the lymph node and traffic back to the site of infection to eradicate virally infected cells. Although most of these effector T cells will undergo apoptosis when the virus is eradicated, a fraction of these cells become long-lived memory cells.[5] On reinfection, the virus-specific memory T cells that were generated from the primary infection will begin to reactivate. Effector memory T cells, which are characterized by their shortened telomeres and lack of CD62L, CD27, and CCR7, are the first responders to antigen.[7,8] T cells can quickly enter nonlymphoid tissue and begin responding to the viral infection. Central memory T cells, on the other hand, do express the adhesion molecules CD62L, CD27, and CCR7 on their surface, and as a result are able to quickly move to lymphoid tissues where their specific antigen is present.[7,8] Here they undergo clonal expansion before migrating to the infected peripheral tissue.

Not all of the antigen-specific CD4+ T cells will migrate to the infected tissue. Activated CD4+ T cells enhance B-cell activation and are necessary for antibody responses to protein antigens.[9,10] B cells receive their first activation signals by follicular DCs or free antigen within the lymphoid follicle.[9,11] On receiving this activation signal, they migrate to the T-cell zone of the lymph node where they come into contact with CD4+ T cells. The T and B cells interact, and the B cells are stimulated by CD40L on the CD4+ T cells and by cytokines. The B cells then migrate back to the germinal center of the lymphoid follicle where they develop into long-lived antibody-producing cells, called plasma cells, or into memory B cells. The plasma and memory forms of B cells are responsible for the protective antibody response that is induced by vaccines, due to their prolonged production of neutralizing antibodies. These antibodies are typically of the IgG isotype.[9,11] Ultimately, it is the level of protective antibody within circulation that determines resistance or susceptibility to the target microbe. As a result, studies assessing the impact of psychosocial stress on vaccination have primarily focused on circulating levels of protective antibodies.

Psychosocial Stressors and Impact on Immunization

One of the central questions regarding psychoneuroimmunology (PNI) is whether exposure to stressors, or certain emotional characteristics or states like anxiety or depression, influence susceptibility and resistance to infectious pathogens. While not feasible for many researchers, experimental infection with live, replicating pathogens can provide important information regarding the impact of emotions on the functioning of the immune system. Studies conducted by Dr Sheldon Cohen and his colleagues have assessed immune responses to viral infection in healthy humans. Subjects were intranasally challenged with different types of respiratory viruses, including rhinovirus, respiratory syncytial virus, corona virus, and influenza A virus.[12] Overall, the studies indicated that symptom severity and the duration of illness tends to be strongest in individuals with higher levels of perceived stress. For example, persons with higher levels of perceived stress produced more nasal mucus after the experimental infection and had higher levels of interleukin (IL)-6 in the nasal secretions, which would reflect a more severe infection.[12] Of note, this effect was dependent on social modifiers. Individuals that were more socially integrated were less likely to develop symptoms from the experimental viral challenge than were individuals that were less socially integrated.[12]

While much can be learned from this type of study, this approach is not feasible for many investigators in PNI, and determining links with subtle psychosocial factors are difficult because of the limited number of subjects that can be challenged with infectious virus. As a result, investigators have begun studying the immune response to different types of vaccines to ultimately understand how psychosocial factors can influence the development of adaptive immunity to microbial challenge.

Designing vaccine-based studies of stress in adults can be difficult because in developed countries, such as the United States, most vaccines are given during childhood. Thus, most participants in laboratory studies already have preexisting immunity to available vaccines, which makes experimental design and data interpretation difficult. Some vaccines, however, have only recently been recommended for children, such as the hepatitis B vaccine. Other vaccines, such as the influenza virus vaccine, vary from year to year based on the analysis of the latest antigenic characteristics of the virus determined by the Centers for Disease Control.[13,14] As a result, many healthy adults are seronegative for hepatitis B and have not generated antigen-specific immunity to the current year's influenza virus vaccines. Thus, these vaccines are useful in assessing how psychosocial factors can influence the development of protective immunity.

Clinical Studies of Stressor Exposure and Vaccination

One of the first studies to demonstrate that exposure to stressful situations would affect the antibody response to vaccines was conducted in medical students who were vaccinated with the recombinant hepatitis B vaccine series.[15] For this vaccine, repeated injections are normally needed to develop protective immunity. In the medical students, approximately 21% developed a protective antibody response after the first vaccine injection, whereas the remaining students developed a protective antibody response after the second injection. Of note, the 21% of the students that seroconverted 1 month after the primary exposure had lower Profile of Mood State anxiety scores than did the students that needed a booster injection to develop protective antibody.[15] This study suggested that mood could significantly change responsiveness to vaccination. Subsequent studies focused more closely on populations experiencing long-term stressful situations.

One such stressful situation is caring for a spouse with a chronic, debilitating illness such as Alzheimer disease. Thus, studies have investigated whether caregivers of spouses with Alzheimer disease develop protective immunity to the influenza vaccine.[16] In comparison with healthy age-matched control subjects, caregivers had lower levels of total and neutralizing antibody to influenza A virus vaccine. This effect could be due to a lack of CD4+ T-cell help, because IL-2 production, which serves to simulate T-cell proliferation, was significantly reduced in the caregivers.[16] The effects of caregiving are not limited to immune responsiveness to an influenza vaccine, because similar results were found using the pneumococcal vaccine.[17]

The effects of caregiving on immune reactivity to the influenza vaccine appear to be strongest in the elderly, as studies in younger adults have been mixed. One study assessing antibody responses to influenza vaccine in nonelderly caregivers of spouses with multiple sclerosis failed to find any decrement in protective antibody responses.[18] In a different study, however, parents caring for children with a developmental disability had lower antibody responses to pneumococcal vaccine than did appropriately matched controls.[19] While it is tempting to speculate that the more consistent results in the elderly are caused by an age-related decrement in immunity, it is also possible that the results reflect differences in stress perception by the participants. For example, older spousal caregivers of dementia patients report greater distress than do younger caregivers of spouses with multiple sclerosis.[18] Moreover, psychosocial factors, such as loneliness and depression, may be important variables in influencing the immune response to vaccines because older caregivers report high levels of depression,[20] whereas loneliness and low social integration appears to be associated with lower antibody responses in medical students [15] as well as university freshmen.[21]

Whereas prolonged stressors have consistently been found to reduce antibody responses to vaccination,[22] short-lasting stressors have been found to enhance the antibody response to vaccination. For example, acute mental stress in the form of a paced mental arithmetic task prior to vaccination with the influenza vaccine resulted in higher antibody titers in women, but not in men, when compared with appropriately matched controls.[23] It is not clear why such effects were found only in women, but it is possible that the results reflect differences in cardiovascular responses to the mental arithmetic. For example, participants who had higher blood pressure during the mental arithmetic and delayed diastolic blood pressure recovery were found to have higher antibody levels to influenza vaccine.[24] Similar results have been found with acute exercise in healthy adults, which has been shown to enhance antibody responses to influenza vaccine in women, and measures of cell-mediated immunity to vaccination in men.[25] This finding has led some to propose exercise as an appropriate behavioral adjuvant to vaccination,[26] which may be particularly important for older individuals. For example, studies have shown that exercise in previously sedentary older individuals significantly increased influenza antibody titers on vaccination.[27] This effect is likely caused by the stimulatory effects of exercise on cell-mediated and humoral immunity, which are often decreased in older individuals.[28,29]

Clinical studies involving human subjects have clearly indicated that psychosocial factors influence the immune response to vaccination. However, these studies have not provided insight into the mechanisms by which psychosocial stressors affect adaptive immunity. The use of animal models has broadened and deepened our understanding of the behavioral and biologic mechanisms by which psychosocial factors affect the immune response. It is somewhat ironic that although most clinical studies of stress and vaccination have assessed neutralizing antibodies to the vaccines, much more is known about stressor-induced modulation of CD8+ T-cell responses in mice. This fact potentially has significant implications for the design of new vaccines, because many current human vaccines do not elicit strong CD8+ T-cell responses. Thus, revealing the underlying stressor-induced mechanisms that alter antiviral CD8+ T-cell responses can lead to the improvement of cell-mediated vaccination strategies. The following discussion highlights some of the important findings in rodent models that provide insight into the mechanisms of neuroendocrine-mediated regulation of antiviral immune function and vaccine efficacy.

Animal Studies Involving Stressor Exposure and Adaptive Immunity

Although not strongly enhanced by many current vaccines, the primary effector cell responsible for eradicating virally infected cells is the cytotoxic CD8+ T cell. The main effector mechanism of CD8+ T cells during a viral infection is the secretion of cytotoxic factors, including cytokines, perforin, and granzymes, that directly mediate the lysis and apoptosis of virally infected cells.[30–33] In addition to the generation of effector responses, successful activation of primary CD8+ T cells in response to antigenic challenge leads to the development of antigen (Ag)-specific memory CD8+ T cells. This process is not only important for the development of memory during an infection but also important for the development of memory responses elicited by vaccination.[34–36] To mount a successful primary adaptive immune response to viral infection, CD8+ T cells must recognize their cognate antigen in the context of MHCI. Antigen-presenting cells, particularly DCs, play a critical role in driving adaptive immune responses, as they both present antigen and present important regulatory signals (eg, costimulatory molecules and cytokines) to T cells during antigen presentation.[37] Both CD8+ T cells and DCs contain receptors for neuroendocrine hormones,[38] therefore neuroendocrine mediators may directly affect CD8+ T cells or may indirectly affect the CD8+ T-cell response by influencing the capability of DCs to take up, process, and present antigen to the T cell.

These mechanisms have been explored in several studies of mice exposed to a prolonged restraint stressor during viral infection with influenza A virus or herpes simplex virus-1 (HSV-1) infection. Restraint is a commonly used murine stressor that induces a consistent and prolonged endocrine stress response, and studies using prolonged restraint found that stressor-induced adrenal glucocorticoid hormones can impair CD8+ T-cell responses to HSV-1.[39–44] Glucocorticoids, namely corticosterone (CORT) in mice and cortisol in humans, are known to decrease nuclear factor-κB activation.[45] This decrease results in the reduction of inflammatory cytokine production and subsequently leads to significant functional consequences in affected cell subsets. Both primary CD8+ T-cell responses as well as the generation of CD8+ T-cell memory responses following vaccination were diminished after exposure to endogenous or exogenous CORT.[41,42] Of importance, the frequency of HSV-specific CD8+ T cells in secondary lymphoid tissues and at the site of HSV infection was significantly reduced; HSV viral titers were increased, and viral clearance was reduced as a consequence of stressor exposure.[39,40] In addition, CD8+ T cells in lymphoid tissue had a reduction in functional capacity as secretion of interferon-γ and granzymes were diminished in stressed mice after HSV infection.[39,40,43,44] This decreased functional capacity translated to weakened protective immunologic memory.[46]

The effects of the stressor on antiviral CD8+ T-cell responses to viral infection were found to be mediated by CORT; administration of the GC receptor antagonist RU486 before and during the stressor restored the number of CD8+ T cells in the lymph nodes of stressor exposed mice.[47] The effects on T cells, however, appear to be indirect, because a study using mice that lack functional GC receptors in their T cells still found that stressor exposure decreased CD8+ T-cell number and function.[43] This result suggested the CORT was not directly inhibiting the CD8+ T cells and suggested that other mechanisms, such as disruption of DC function or reduced CD4+ T-cell help, were at play. Consistent with this view, DC function was found to be significantly impaired by CORT, which was associated with a decrease in antigen-specific CD8+

T-cell proliferation.[43] In vitro, it was shown that CORT disrupts the ability of DCs to process and present viral antigens to T cells,[48,49] ultimately suggesting that stressor-induced CORT decreases the ability of DCs to present antigen and stimulate CD8+ T-cell function. Although these studies were focused on CD8+ T cells, because DCs also activate CD4+ T cells and B cells,[37] CORT-induced suppression of DC function likely affects CD4+ T-cell activity and B-cell antibody production.

Other neuroendocrine mediators have been shown to play an important role in immune regulation during the stress response. In mice exposed to the prolonged restraint stressor and subsequently infected with influenza A, it was evident that blocking GC receptors alone did not restore all of the stress-induced changes of the immune system.[50–53] While blocking GC receptors reversed the stress-induced decrease in leukocyte trafficking into lymphoid tissues and the lungs, the function of these cells was not restored.[51] Of note, blocking the effects of stressor-induced catecholamines (ie, epinephrine and norepinephrine) by antagonizing β-adrenergic receptors during stress restored the activation of CD8+ T lymphocytes in stressor-exposed mice challenged with influenza virus.[51] In several studies a chemical sympathectomy with 6-hydroxydopamine prior to infection resulted in alteration in primary and memory CD8+ T-cell responses.[54,55] These studies in rodents, as well as many other laboratory animal studies, demonstrate the many, and complex, ways through which psychological stressors affect the immune response.

Human clinical studies assessing the impact of stressor exposure on the immune response to vaccines show that while some stressors, such as caregiving, tend to decrease the adaptive immune response, acute stressors tend to enhance adaptive immunity. Similar differences are evident with animal stressors, and a study by Powell and colleagues[56] showed that DCs from mice exposed to a repeated social stressor have an increase in costimulatory molecules important for CD8+ T-cell activation (eg, CD80, MHCI, CD44) on their cell surface and secrete an increased amount of inflammatory cytokines in response to in vitro stimulation of Toll-like receptors. Repeated exposure to social stress has also been shown to enhance the adaptive response to influenza virus infection, by increasing the number of antigen-specific memory CD8+ T cells that are critical for establishing virus-specific immunologic memory.[57] Together, these studies suggest that the stressor enhanced the ability of the DCs to process antigen and stimulate adaptive immunity. Although it is not completely clear why this stressor would enhance, rather than suppress, DC activity, it was shown that exposure to the social stressor caused the DC to be resistant to the suppressive effects of CORT.[56] These studies indicate that when determining the impact of stressor-induced hormones on adaptive immunity, a crucial mediating factor is the impact that the hormones have on antigen-presenting cells. Whether stressors enhance or suppress antigen-presenting cell activity likely determines whether stressor exposure will enhance or suppress the immune response to vaccination.

SUMMARY

There is now ample evidence that psychosocial factors affect the immune response to vaccination. For the most part, studies have found that prolonged, life-altering stressors, such as caring for a spouse with a chronic and debilitating illness, decrease the antibody response to vaccination. Although less well studied, this effect is likely caused by stress perception and available coping resources, because factors such as perceived burden, loneliness, and social support have been found to be associated with the altered immune response. The impact of stressor exposure on immune responses to vaccines can also be enhancive, but in this case the stressor tends to be in the form of an acute, short-lasting stressor. Exercise in previously sedentary adults has also been shown to boost the immune response, making it an intriguing possible adjuvant to vaccination.

While human studies continue to define stressor characteristics and psychosocial variables that lead to immunosuppression versus immunoenhancement, very little is known regarding the biologic mechanisms through which stressors affect the immune response to vaccines. Studies in laboratory animals, however, have found that stressor-induced hormones affect the ability of antigen-presenting cells, primarily DCs, to process and present viral antigen. The primary mediating hormone appears to be CORT. Stressors that cause a prolonged increase in CORT, such as prolonged restraint, suppress the ability of DCs to process and present antigen, and stressors that induce DC resistance to CORT, such as social stress, increase the ability of DCs to process and present antigen. These effects on the DC significantly affect the development of antigen-specific memory T cells, and although less well studied, are also likely to affect the antibody response to vaccines. As research progresses in both humans and laboratory animals, the complete set of psychological and physiological factors by which stressor exposure affects the immune response to vaccines will become more clearly defined.

REFERENCES

1. Ten great public health achievements—United States, 1900–1999. MMWR Morb Mortal Wkly Rep 1999;48(12):241–3.
2. Stern AM, Markel H. The history of vaccines and immunization: familiar patterns, new challenges. Health Aff (Millwood) 2005;24(3):611–21.
3. Hill DJ, Griffiths NJ, Borodina E, et al. Cellular and molecular biology of *Neisseria meningitidis* colonization and invasive disease. Clin Sci (Lond) 2010;118(9): 547–64.
4. McMurry JA, Johansson BE, De Groot AS. A call to cellular & humoral arms: enlisting cognate T cell help to develop broad-spectrum vaccines against influenza A. Hum Vaccin 2008;4(2):148–57.
5. Cox RJ, Brokstad KA, Ogra P. Influenza virus: immunity and vaccination strategies. Comparison of the immune response to inactivated and live, attenuated influenza vaccines. Scand J Immunol 2004;59(1):1–15.
6. La Gruta NL, Kedzierska K, Stambas J, et al. A question of self-preservation: immunopathology in influenza virus infection. Immunol Cell Biol 2007;85(2):85–92.
7. Wherry EJ, Teichgraber V, Becker TC, et al. Lineage relationship and protective immunity of memory CD8 T cell subsets. Nat Immunol 2003;4(3):225–34.
8. Willinger T, Freeman T, Hasegawa H, et al. Molecular signatures distinguish human central memory from effector memory CD8 T cell subsets. J Immunol 2005;175(9):5895–903.
9. Baumgarth N. Nicole Baumgarth: tackling flu from a B cell angle. interviewed by Amy Maxmem. J Exp Med 2008;205(11):2454–5.
10. McKinstry KK, Strutt TM, Swain SL. The potential of CD4 T-cell memory. Immunology 2010;130(1):1–9.
11. Baumgarth N, Choi YS, Rothaeusler K, et al. B cell lineage contributions to antiviral host responses. Curr Top Microbiol Immunol 2008;31941–61.
12. Cohen S. Keynote presentation at the Eighth International Congress of Behavioral Medicine: the Pittsburgh common cold studies: psychosocial predictors of susceptibility to respiratory infectious illness. Int J Behav Med 2005;12(3):123–31.

13. Fiore AE, Shay DK, Broder K, et al. Prevention and control of seasonal influenza with vaccines: recommendations of the advisory committee on immunization practices (ACIP), 2009. MMWR Recomm Rep 2009;58(RR-8):1–52.
14. Russell CA, Jones TC, Barr IG, et al. Influenza vaccine strain selection and recent studies on the global migration of seasonal influenza viruses. Vaccine 2008; 26(Suppl 4):D31–4.
15. Glaser R, Kiecolt-Glaser JK, Bonneau RH, et al. Stress-induced modulation of the immune response to recombinant hepatitis B vaccine. Psychosom Med 1992; 54(1):22–9.
16. Kiecolt-Glaser JK, Glaser R, Gravenstein S, et al. Chronic stress alters the immune response to influenza virus vaccine in older adults. Proc Natl Acad Sci U S A 1996;93(7):3043–7.
17. Glaser R, Sheridan J, Malarkey WB, et al. Chronic stress modulates the immune response to a pneumococcal pneumonia vaccine. Psychosom Med 2000;62(6): 804–7.
18. Vedhara K, McDermott MP, Evans TG, et al. Chronic stress in nonelderly caregivers: psychological, endocrine and immune implications. J Psychosom Res 2002;53(6):1153–61.
19. Gallagher S, Phillips AC, Drayson MT, et al. Caregiving for children with developmental disabilities is associated with a poor antibody response to influenza vaccination. Psychosom Med 2009;71(3):341–4.
20. Pinquart M, Sorensen S. Associations of stressors and uplifts of caregiving with caregiver burden and depressive mood: a meta-analysis. J Gerontol B Psychol Sci Soc Sci 2003;58(2):112–28.
21. Pressman SD, Cohen S, Miller GE, et al. Loneliness, social network size, and immune response to influenza vaccination in college freshmen. Health Psychol 2005;24(3):297–306.
22. Pedersen AF, Zachariae R, Bovbjerg DH. Psychological stress and antibody response to influenza vaccination: a meta-analysis. Brain Behav Immun 2009; 23(4):427–33.
23. Edwards KM, Burns VE, Reynolds T, et al. Acute stress exposure prior to influenza vaccination enhances antibody response in women. Brain Behav Immun 2006;20(2):159–68.
24. Phillips AC, Carroll D, Burns VE, et al. Cardiovascular activity and the antibody response to vaccination. J Psychosom Res 2009;67(1):37–43.
25. Edwards KM, Burns VE, Allen LM, et al. Eccentric exercise as an adjuvant to influenza vaccination in humans. Brain Behav Immun 2007;21(2):209–17.
26. Edwards KM, Campbell JP, Ring C, et al. Exercise intensity does not influence the efficacy of eccentric exercise as a behavioural adjuvant to vaccination. Brain Behav Immun 2010;24(4):623–30.
27. Woods JA, Keylock KT, Lowder T, et al. Cardiovascular exercise training extends influenza vaccine seroprotection in sedentary older adults: the immune function intervention trial. J Am Geriatr Soc 2009;57(12):2183–91.
28. Haaland DA, Sabljic TF, Baribeau DA, et al. Is regular exercise a friend or foe of the aging immune system? a systematic review. Clin J Sport Med 2008;18(6): 539–48.
29. Yan H, Kuroiwa A, Tanaka H, et al. Effect of moderate exercise on immune senescence in men. Eur J Appl Physiol 2001;86(2):105–11.
30. Doherty PC. Cell mediated immunity in virus infections. Biosci Rep 1997;17(4): 367–87.

31. Doherty PC, Hamilton-Easton AM, Topham DJ, et al. Consequences of viral infections for lymphocyte compartmentalization and homeostasis. Semin Immunol 1997;9(6):365–73.

32. Doherty PC, Riberdy JM, Belz GT. Quantitative analysis of the CD8+ T-cell response to readily eliminated and persistent viruses. Philos Trans R Soc Lond, B, Biol Sci 2000;355(1400):1093–101.

33. Lukacher AE, Braciale VL, Braciale TJ. In vivo effector function of influenza virus-specific cytotoxic T lymphocyte clones is highly specific. J Exp Med 1984;160(3):814–26.

34. Welsh RM, Selin LK, Szomolanyi-Tsuda E. Immunological memory to viral infections. Annu Rev Immunol 2004;22711–43.

35. Wong P, Lara-Tejero M, Ploss A, et al. Rapid development of T cell memory. J Immunol 2004;172(12):7239–45.

36. Wong P, Pamer EG. CD8 T cell responses to infectious pathogens. Annu Rev Immunol 2003;2129–70.

37. Banchereau J, Briere F, Caux C, et al. Immunobiology of dendritic cells. Annu Rev Immunol 2000;18767–811.

38. Bailey M, Engler H, Hunzeker J, et al. The hypothalamic-pituitary-adrenal axis and viral infection. Viral Immunol 2003;16(2):141–57.

39. Ashcraft KA, Bonneau RH. Psychological stress exacerbates primary vaginal herpes simplex virus type 1 (HSV-1) infection by impairing both innate and adaptive immune responses. Brain Behav Immun 2008;22(8):1231–40.

40. Ashcraft KA, Hunzeker J, Bonneau RH. Psychological stress impairs the local CD8+ T cell response to mucosal HSV-1 infection and allows for increased pathogenicity via a glucocorticoid receptor-mediated mechanism. Psychoneuroendocrinology 2008;33(7):951–63.

41. Bonneau RH, Sheridan JF, Feng NG, et al. Stress-induced effects on cell-mediated innate and adaptive memory components of the murine immune response to herpes simplex virus infection. Brain Behav Immun 1991;5(3):274–95.

42. Bonneau RH, Sheridan JF, Feng NG, et al. Stress-induced suppression of herpes simplex virus (HSV)-specific cytotoxic T lymphocyte and natural killer cell activity and enhancement of acute pathogenesis following local HSV infection. Brain Behav Immun 1991;5(2):170–92.

43. Elftman MD, Hunzeker JT, Mellinger JC, et al. Stress-induced glucocorticoids at the earliest stages of herpes simplex virus-1 infection suppress subsequent antiviral immunity, implicating impaired dendritic cell function. J Immunol 2010; 184(4):1867–75.

44. Freeman ML, Sheridan BS, Bonneau RH, et al. Psychological stress compromises CD8+ T cell control of latent herpes simplex virus type 1 infections. J Immunol 2007;179(1):322–8.

45. Padgett DA, Glaser R. How stress influences the immune response. Trends Immunol 2003;24(8):444–8.

46. Wonnacott KM, Bonneau RH. The effects of stress on memory cytotoxic T lymphocyte-mediated protection against herpes simplex virus infection at mucosal sites. Brain Behav Immun 2002;16(2):104–17.

47. Nair A, Hunzeker J, Bonneau RH. Modulation of microglia and CD8(+) T cell activation during the development of stress-induced herpes simplex virus type-1 encephalitis. Brain Behav Immun 2007;21(6):791–806.

48. Truckenmiller ME, Bonneau RH, Norbury CC. Stress presents a problem for dendritic cells: corticosterone and the fate of MHC class I antigen processing and presentation. Brain Behav Immun 2006;20(3):210–8.

49. Truckenmiller ME, Princiotta MF, Norbury CC, et al. Corticosterone impairs MHC class I antigen presentation by dendritic cells via reduction of peptide generation. J Neuroimmunol 2005;160(1–2):48–60.

50. Hermann G, Beck FM, Sheridan JF. Stress-induced glucocorticoid response modulates mononuclear cell trafficking during an experimental influenza viral infection. J Neuroimmunol 1995;56(2):179–86.

51. Hermann G, Beck FM, Tovar CA, et al. Stress-induced changes attributable to the sympathetic nervous system during experimental influenza viral infection in DBA/2 inbred mouse strain. J Neuroimmunol 1994;53(2):173–80.

52. Hermann G, Tovar CA, Beck FM, et al. Restraint stress differentially affects the pathogenesis of an experimental influenza viral infection in three inbred strains of mice. J Neuroimmunol 1993;47(1):83–94.

53. Hermann G, Tovar CA, Beck FM, et al. Kinetics of glucocorticoid response to restraint stress and/or experimental influenza viral infection in two inbred strains of mice. J Neuroimmunol 1994;49(1–2):25–33.

54. Grebe KM, Takeda K, Hickman HD, et al. Cutting edge: sympathetic nervous system increases proinflammatory cytokines and exacerbates influenza a virus pathogenesis. J Immunol 2010;184(2):540–4.

55. Leo NA, Callahan TA, Bonneau RH. Peripheral sympathetic denervation alters both the primary and memory cellular immune responses to herpes simplex virus infection. Neuroimmunomodulation 1998;5(1–2):22–35.

56. Powell ND, Bailey MT, Mays JW, et al. Repeated social defeat activates dendritic cells and enhances Toll-like receptor dependent cytokine secretion. Brain Behav Immun 2009;23(2):225–31.

57. Mays JW, Bailey MT, Hunzeker JT, et al. Influenza virus-specific immunological memory is enhanced by repeated social defeat. J Immunol 2010;184(4):2014–25.

The Impact of Psychological Stress on Wound Healing: Methods and Mechanisms

Jean-Philippe Gouin, MA[a,b,*], Janice K. Kiecolt-Glaser, PhD[a,b,c]

KEYWORDS

- Wound healing • Stress • Cytokine • Cortisol
- Psychoneuroimmunology • Oxytocin

Wound healing is a critical process involved in the recovery from injury and surgical procedures. Poor healing increases the risk for wound infections or complications, lengthens hospital stays, magnifies patient discomfort, and slows return to activities of daily living. Converging evidence from different research paradigms suggests that psychological stress and other behavioral factors can affect wound healing. A meta-analytical study using diverse wound-healing models and outcomes found that across studies there was an average correlation of -0.42 between psychological stress and wound healing.[1] This result suggests that the relationship between stress and wound repair is not only statistically significant but also clinically relevant. This review presents data and methods from observational, experimental, and interventional studies corroborating the impact of stress on wound healing. Potential behavioral and physiologic mechanisms explaining the association between stress and impaired wound healing are also discussed.

Work on this article was supported by a doctoral research training award from the Fonds de la Recherche en Santé du Québec and NIH grants AG029562, CA126857, CA131029, AT003912, Ohio State Comprehensive Cancer Center Core Grant CA16058, and NCRR Grant UL1RR025755.
[a] Department of Psychology, The Ohio State University, 225 Psychology Building, 1835 Neil Avenue, Columbus, OH 43210, USA
[b] Institute for Behavioral Medicine Research, The Ohio State University College of Medicine, 460 Medical Center Drive, Room 139, Columbus, OH 43210-1228, USA
[c] Department of Psychiatry, The Ohio State University College of Medicine, 1670 Upham Drive, Columbus, OH 43210, USA
* Corresponding author. Institute for Behavioral Medicine Research, The Ohio State University College of Medicine, 460 Medical Center Drive, Room 139, Columbus, OH 43210-1228.
E-mail address: Gouin.1@osu.edu

OBSERVATIONAL STUDIES

Prospective studies examining wound healing–related complications following surgery provide evidence for the impact of stress on wound repair. Greater fear or distress before surgery has been associated with poorer outcomes including longer hospital stays, more postoperative complications, and higher rates of rehospitalization.[2,3] For example, among 111 patients undergoing gallstone removal surgery, those who reported more stress on the third postoperative day had a longer hospital stay, compared with less anxious individuals.[4] Among 309 consenting consecutive patients who underwent an elective coronary artery bypass graft surgery, patients who were more optimistic were less likely to be re-hospitalized than less optimistic individuals. Conversely, patients who experienced more depressive symptoms were more likely to require rehospitalization for infection-related complications than individuals reporting less distress.[5] This result was replicated in a study of 72 patients undergoing coronary artery bypass surgery. Patient who had more depressive symptoms at discharge had more infections and poorer wound healing in the following 6 weeks after surgery than participants who reported less distress.[6]

Psychological factors can also modulate healing of chronic wounds. Fifty-three older adults with chronic lower leg wounds were followed longitudinally to assess speed of wound repair. Patients who experienced the highest levels of depression and anxiety (based on a median split of the Hospital Anxiety and Depression Scale) were 4 times more likely to be categorized in the delayed healing group than individuals who reported less distress.[7] Of importance, in these observational studies distress predicted wound-healing outcomes over and above differences in sociodemographic variables and medical status. Psychological distress thus appears to influence recovery from medical procedures and healing of chronic wounds in clinical settings.

EXPERIMENTAL STUDIES

Animal and human studies in which standard wounds are created experimentally and healing is closely monitored over time provide the strongest evidence of the impact of stress on wound repair. Three main wounding methodologies have been used to study the effect of stress on wound healing.

Punch Biopsy Model

Punch biopsies are used to create standard full-thickness dermal wounds as well as mucosal wounds. Daily pictures of the wound allow for a quantification of changes in wound size over time.

The first human experimental study that examined the impact of stress on wound healing involved family dementia caregivers. Caregivers have to deal daily with the loss of memory, inappropriate emotions, and wandering and restless behavior of their loved ones. Caregiving stress has been associated with heightened anxiety and depression, immune dysregulation, increased risk for cardiovascular disorders, and even death.[8] Family dementia caregiving thus represents an excellent model of chronic stress in humans. A 3.5-mm punch biopsy wound was created on the nondominant forearm of 13 women caregivers and 13 sociodemographically similar noncaregiving controls. Caregivers took 24% longer to heal the small, standardized dermal wound than matched controls, providing initial evidence that chronic stress can delay wound repair.[9]

Stress can also impede healing of a punch biopsy wound among younger people who experienced less intense stress. Twenty-four healthy young men were followed for 21 days after a standard 4-mm punch biopsy was performed on their forearm. In that study, wound healing was assessed using ultrasound biomicroscopy. Stress levels were measured using a self-report questionnaire, the Perceived Stress Scale. Higher perceived stress on the day of the biopsy was associated with slower wound healing.[10] A substantial correlation of −0.59 was found between perceived stress and healing progress between the days 7 and 21 after the biopsy.[10]

Pain, a physical and psychological stressor, can also influence wound healing. A 2-mm full-thickness wound was placed on the back of one upper arm of obese women before receiving elective gastric bypass surgery. Greater acute pain immediately after surgery and persistent pain in the 4 weeks following surgery were associated with slower healing of the experimental wound.[11] Pain generates psychological distress and, when compounded by the presence of other stressors, can put a person at increased risk for delayed wound repair.[12]

Well-controlled animal studies corroborate the impact of stress on wound healing observed in humans. Mice subjected to restraint stress healed a standardized 3.5-mm full-thickness punch biopsy wound on average of 27% more slowly than control mice who were not exposed to the stressor.[13] Restraint stress was also associated with delayed wound healing in a reptilian species, *Urosaurus ornatus* (tree lizard).[14] Social stressors can also impair wound healing. Monogamous California mice, *Peromyscus californicus*, healed a punch biopsy wound more slowly when stressed by the separation from their conspecifics, compared with when they were continuously housed with their conspecifics.[15]

Like cutaneous wounds, mucosal wound healing is also responsive to psychological stress, as demonstrated by a study with academic examination stress. Using a within-subject design, 11 dental students had a biopsy performed on their hard palate during their summer vacation and again 3 days before a major examination. Mucosal wounds placed before the examination healed on average 40% more slowly than identical wounds made during summer vacation. Of importance, the differences in the rate of healing were very consistent: no student healed as rapidly during examinations as during vacation.[16]

The impact of negative emotions on mucosal wound healing was replicated in a larger study. Among 193 healthy undergraduate students who received a 3.5-mm wound on the hard palate, individuals reporting high levels of depressive symptoms were almost 3.6 times more likely to be classified as slow healers than less dysphoric students.[17]

Blister Wounds Model

The blister wounds model is another experimental paradigm designed to study the impact of psychological factors on wound healing. Blister wounds are produced by the application of a vacuum pump on the forearm. A gentle suction creates a separation of the epidermis from the dermis over the course of 1 hour. One of the strengths of this method is that it allows for the collection of data on cytokine production at the wound site, as described below. In this model, wound healing is assessed via measurement of the rate of transepidermal water loss (TEWL). One of the main functions of the skin is to limit movement of water in and out of the body. The permeability of the epidermis increases after the blister wound, but decreases as the healing process unfolds. A computerized evaporimetry instrument can measure vapor pressure gradient in the air layers close to the skin surface. TEWL measurement is a noninvasive means to monitor changes in the stratum corneum barrier function of the skin that provides an excellent objective method for the evaluation of wound healing.

Using a blister wounds paradigm, the discussion of a marital disagreement, a commonplace stressor, delayed wound repair. Married couples were invited for two 24-hour admissions at a hospital research unit. During both visits, 8 8-mm suction blisters were created on the participants' nondominant forearm. Wound healing was monitored for 14 days using TEWL measurements. During the first admission, couples participated in a structured social support interaction task. During the second visit, couples were asked to discuss marital disagreements during a 30-minute period. After both interaction tasks, couples remained in the research unit until the next morning to allow for cytokine measurements and to minimize external influences on wound healing.[18]

Couples' blister wounds healed more slowly following the marital conflict visit than after the social support visit, suggesting that the stress induced by the discussion of marital disagreements interfered with wound repair. Furthermore, the quality of the discussion also influenced the rate of healing. Couples who had more hostile and negative interactions across both the support and the conflict discussions healed wounds more slowly than couples whose interactions were less negative. The overall differences related to hostility were substantial. The blister wounds in high hostile couples healed at only 60% of the rate of low hostile couples.[18]

In a different subset of participants from the same study, positive behaviors during the social support task were also related to wound repair. Individuals who displayed more self-disclosure, acceptance of their partner, relationship-enhancing statements, and humor during the interaction task healed the blister wounds faster than participants who exhibited less positive behaviors during the marital interaction task.[19]

Difficulties in managing one's anger has also been associated with impaired wound healing. Blister wounds were created on the forearm of 98 community-dwelling participants who were followed for 14 days to monitor healing speed. Anger management styles were assessed via a self-report questionnaire, the Spielberger Anger Expression Scale. Participants who had difficulty controlling the expression of their anger were 4.2 times more likely to be classified as slow healers than individuals who reported better anger control. Furthermore, individuals with anger management issues secreted more cortisol in response to the blistering procedure. The increased glucocorticoid production was in turn related to delayed healing.[20]

Tape Stripping to Disrupt Skin Barrier Function

Another wound-healing model consists of the repeated application of cellophane tape to remove a layer of epidermis cells, causing a disruption of the stratum corneum barrier function of the skin. This procedure affects epidermal permeability. Wound healing is assessed by measuring the rate of recovery of the skin barrier function using TEWL measurements.

Acute laboratory stressors can delay the recovery of skin barrier function following its disruption by tape stripping. Twenty-five women participated in the Trier Social Stress Test (TSST), a psychosical stressor.[21] The TSST, a standardized laboratory stressor with a mock job interview and a mental arithmetic task, induces reliable changes in heart rate, and cortisol and cytokine production, and subjective anxiety responses.[22,23] Skin barrier repair was delayed in women after the TSST as compared with a stress-free period.[21]

This result was replicated in a larger study of 85 healthy young men and women. Individuals who participated in the TSST had a slower recovery of skin barrier function than participants who engaged in a reading control task.[24] Furthermore, positive affect had a protective effect on stress-induced delays in skin barrier recovery. Stressed individuals reporting more positive affect recovered faster from the tape-stripping procedure than stressed participants who had low-trait positive affect.[25]

Academic examination stress affects skin barrier recovery. Twenty-seven professional and medical students underwent a tape stripping procedure on 3 occasions: right after their winter and spring vacations, and during their winter final examination week. Skin barrier recovery was significantly delayed at 3, 6, and 24 hours after tape stripping during the examination period, compared with the 2 vacation periods. Furthermore, students reporting the most stress during the examination period had slower recovery in skin barrier function than participants who experienced less examination-induced stress.[26]

The interpersonal stress associated with the dissolution of a committed marital relationship can impede recovery of the stratum corneum barrier function of the skin. Twenty-eight women who were going through a divorce or a separation and 27 women who reported high levels of marital satisfaction underwent a tape-stripping procedure on both facial cheeks. Socially stressed women had delayed skin barrier recovery at 3 and 24 hours following the tape-stripping procedure, compared with less stressed women.[27]

In animal models, different types of stressors can also impair skin barrier recovery. Three days of immobilization stress delayed skin barrier function recovery even for 7 days, compared with control rats not exposed to the stressor.[28] Social reorganization stress associated with cage transfer also impaired the restoration of skin barrier function in rats.[29] These results converge with human data indicating that psychological stress can disrupt skin barrier recovery.

INTERVENTION STUDIES

Intervention studies that improve healing outcomes by reducing psychological stress provide further evidence of the impact of psychological and behavioral factors in wound repair. Meta-analyses of clinical studies show that behavioral stress management interventions before surgery have been associated with improved postoperative outcomes, including fewer medical complications and shorter hospital stays.[30,31]

Written emotional disclosure interventions can decrease psychological distress, improve self-reported health, enhance aspects of cellular immunity, and decrease health care use.[32] Men were randomized to a written emotional disclosure intervention or a nonintervention control group, and received a punch biopsy on the nondominant forearm. Healing was assessed using ultrasound biomicroscopy on 3 occasions during a 21-day period. Men who participated in the emotional disclosure intervention had smaller wounds than control participants at 14 and 21 days.[33]

Physical exercise can reduce psychological distress in addition to improving cardiovascular function.[34] Older adults were randomized to an exercise intervention (1-hour aerobic exercise session, 3 times per week) or a nonintervention control group. One month after the beginning of the intervention, participants received a 3.5-mm punch biopsy on the back of their nondominant upper arm. Older adults who exercised healed their wounds faster than those in the control group.[35] In accord with these human data, older mice randomized to a 30-minute daily exercise period during 8 days healed a punch biopsy wound faster than sedentary control mice.[36]

Social support is associated with better health outcomes.[37] In animal studies, monogamous rodents who were housed in pairs healed a standard punch biopsy wound faster than rodents housed alone.[38] Pair housing also buffered the impact of restraint stress on wound healing. Immobilization stress impaired cutaneous wound healing in Siberian hamsters housed alone, but not in hamsters housed in pairs.[39]

These data indicate that the presence of a familial conspecific improves wound-healing outcomes in monogamous rodents.

A pharmacologic agent commonly used in the treatment of mood and anxiety disorders is fluoxetine.[40] In a study using alternating isolation and crowding stress, stressed Wistar rats who received fluoxetine healed at a similar pace as their nonstress counterparts, and faster than stressed animals who received only a vehicle injection.[41] These results indicate that pharmacologic stress reduction may also improve wound healing.

In summary, a wide array of acute and chronic stressors can disrupt the healing process. Furthermore, the impact of stress on wound repair has been observed across different methodologies and with different healing outcomes, and most results have replicated in at least 2 independent laboratories. Results from observation, experimental, and intervention studies collectively provide strong evidence that psychological stress can influence wound healing.

BIOLOGY OF WOUND HEALING

A brief review of the biology of wound healing is presented to highlight the pathways by which psychological stress can impede the repair process. Wound healing progresses through several overlapping stages.[42] In the initial inflammatory stage, vasoconstriction and blood coagulation are followed by platelet activation and the release of platelet-derived growth factors (PDGFs) as well as chemoattractant factors released by injured parenchymal cells. Cytokines and chemokines, such as interleukin (IL)-1α, IL-1β, transforming growth factor-β (TGF-β), vascular endothelial growth factor, tumor necrosis factor-α (TNF-α), and IL-8 play important roles in the early stage of wound healing. These factors act as chemoattractants for the migration of phagocytes and other cells to the site, starting the proliferative phase that involves the recruitment and replication of cells necessary for tissue regeneration and capillary regrowth. The final step, wound remodeling, may continue for weeks or months. Thus, the healing process is a cascade, and success in the later stages of wound repair is highly dependent on initial events.[42]

Inflammation plays a key role early in this cascade, and proinflammatory cytokines are essential to this effort; they help to protect against infection and prepare injured tissue for repair by enhancing the recruitment and activation of phagocytes.[43] Furthermore, cytokines released by recruited cells regulate the ability of fibroblasts and epithelial cells to remodel the damaged tissue.[43] IL-1 produced early after tissue injury can regulate the production, release, and activation of metalloproteinases that are important in the destruction and remodeling of the wound; IL-1 also regulates fibroblast chemotaxis and the production of collagen.[43] Moreover, IL-1 stimulates the production of other cytokines that are important for wound healing, including IL-2, IL-6, and IL-8.[43] Confirming the importance of proinflammatory cytokines in the healing process, IL-6 knock-out mice healed a standard wound 3 times more slowly than wild-type mice.[44] Accordingly, deficits early in the wound repair cascade can have adverse downstream consequences.

PHYSIOLOGIC PATHWAYS OF THE STRESS-INDUCED WOUND-HEALING IMPAIRMENT

Psychological stress leads to the activation of the hypothalamic-pituitary-adrenal and the sympathetic-adrenal-medullary axes.[45] Enhanced glucocorticoids and catecholamines production can directly influence several components of the healing process. Substantial evidence from animal and humans studies indicate that physiologic stress responses can retard the initial inflammatory phase of wound healing.[46] **Fig. 1**

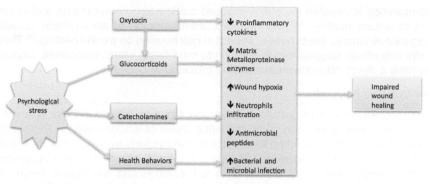

Fig. 1. Behavioral and physiologic pathways linking psychological stress and wound healing.

presents a schematic representation of the behavioral and physiologic pathways linking stress and wound healing.

Glucocorticoids

Stress-induced glucocorticoid production has been associated with delayed wound healing. In humans, greater awakening cortisol secretion the day following a punch biopsy was associated with greater perceived stress and delayed wound healing.[10] In animal studies, restraint stress led to a fourfold elevation in corticosterone levels.[13] Blocking glucocorticoid function with a glucocorticoid receptor antagonist, RU40555, eliminated the stress-induced delay in wound healing in stressed animals.[13,39] Preventing glucocorticoid production via adrenalectomy also reduced the effects of restraint stress on wound healing.[39] Furthermore, exogenous administration of glucocorticoid slowed wound healing as compared with a vehicle injection.[13]

Catecholamines

Increased catecholamine production also appears to play a role in stress-induced impairment in wound healing. Administration of an α-adrenergic receptor antagonist attenuated the restraint stress-induced impairment of wound healing in mice.[47] In a study using a rotation stress model, administration of a β-adrenergic receptor antagonist, propranolol hydrochloride, attenuated the stress-induced impairment in wound healing in mice.[48] In a burn wound model, mice injected with a β-adrenergic receptor antagonist exhibited improved reepithelialization of burn wounds, compared with mice who received a vehicle injection.[49] Furthermore, injection of norepinephrine can reduce keratinocyte motility and migration in vitro.[49] These data provide evidence of a role for catecholamines in stress-induced impairment in wound repair.

Oxytocin and Vasopressin

The two hypothalamic peptides, oxytocin and vasopressin, modulated physiologic stress responses and social bonding processes in animal and human work. In a couples study using the blister wounds model, individuals who had more positive interactions with their partner during a social support task had higher plasma oxytocin levels. Higher circulating oxytocin levels were in turn associated with faster healing of the standard blister wounds. Furthermore, in women, but not in men, greater plasma vasopressin levels were related to faster healing.[19]

Well-controlled animal studies corroborate the role of oxytocin in mediating the beneficial effects of social relationships on wound healing. Exogenous oxytocin administration attenuated the stress-induced corticosterone production and impairment in wound healing.[39,50] Furthermore, administration of an oxytocin receptor antagonist eliminated the beneficial impact of pair housing on wound healing.[39] These results collectively suggest that in addition to modulating stress responses, oxytocin may have a direct influence on the healing process.

Local Cytokine Production

Diminished expression of proinflammatory cytokines at the wound site is another pathway by which stress can delay the initial phase of wound healing. The suction blister model provides a method to monitor in vivo cytokine expression at the wound site in humans. After raising several blisters and removing their roofs (the epidermis), plastic templates with wells containing a salt solution and autologous serum are placed over the lesions to monitor protein expression at the wound site. The autologous serum-buffer solution is aspirated from the wells with a syringe at different time intervals, allowing for cell phenotyping and cytokine measurement as the local immune response evolves.

Using this approach, women who reported more perceived stress produced significantly lower IL-1α and IL-8 levels at the wound site, 5 and 24 hours after the blistering procedure.[51] Marital disagreement also influenced local cytokine production.[18] Production of three proinflammatory cytokines at the wound site, IL-1β, IL-6, and TNF-α, were lower after the discussion of a marital disagreement than after a social support discussion, paralleling the impact of marital conflict on wound healing.[18] In these two studies, local cytokine production was not significantly associated with serum levels of the same cytokines, underscoring the different biologic significance of local and systemic production of these molecules.

In a clinical study, patients undergoing surgery for hernia removal who reported greater preoperative stress had a lower concentration of IL-1β in the wound drain fluid 20 hours after the operation, compared with patients who experienced less preoperative distress.[52] Furthermore, two stressors that can impair cutaneous and mucosal wound healing, family dementia caregiving and academic examinations, were also associated with poorer stimulated production of IL-1β after treatment with lipopolysaccharide.[9,16] Corroborating human data, mice subjected to restraint stress had lower levels of IL-1β mRNA at the wound site, compared with control mice.[53,54]

Stress-induced glucocorticoid production might effectively decrease cytokine production at the wound site. Exogenous administration of glucocorticoid diminished IL-1α, IL-1β, and TNF-α expression at the site after wounding in mice.[42] Similarly, animal and human studies have also demonstrated that stress-induced elevations in glucocorticoids can transiently suppress IL-1β, TNF-α, and PDGF production.[51,54] Accordingly, dysregulation of glucocorticoid secretion provides one obvious neuroendocrine pathway through which stress alters the initial inflammatory phase of wound healing.

Matrix Metalloproteinase

Matrix metalloproteinase (MMP) enzymes are involved in the degradation of collagen and other extracellular matrix molecules. Degradation of the basement membrane of the wound promotes cellular invasion and migration, an essential component of the early phase of wound healing. Among patients undergoing inguinal hernia surgery, those who reported greater worry about the operation had lower levels of MMP-9 in the wound drain fluid 20 hours after surgery.[52] In a human study using the blister wounds model, there was a negative correlation between plasma cortisol levels and MMP-2 protein levels at the wound site.[55] Furthermore, in an animal study using a rotation stress model, mice subjected to the stressor had fewer activated MMP-2 and MMP-9 7 days after wounding, compared with control mice.[48] These data indicate that stress can downregulate MMP production at the wound site.

Wound Cellularity

Psychological stress may reduce cell infiltration at the wound site. In a study using a restraint stress paradigm, cellularity of the wound and wound margin areas were analyzed in cross sections of dermal and epidermal layers. Mice subjected to restraint stress had less leukocyte infiltration to the wound sites than control mice at 1 and 3 days after wounding.[13]

Increased Susceptibility to Infection

Stress can also increase susceptibility to wound infection. Mice exposed to restraint stress had a 2- to 5-log increase in opportunistic bacteria such as *Staphylococcus aureus*, compared with control mice not exposed to the stressor. Furthermore, 7 days after wounding, 85.4% of restraint-stress mice had bacterial counts predictive of infection, compared with 27.4% of controls.[56]

The increased susceptibility to infection appears to be mediated in part by a decreased epidermal antimicrobial peptides production. Mice exposed to insomnia and crowding stress had lower epidermis levels of cathelin-related antimicrobial peptides and exhibited more severe infection following an intradermal injection of group A *Streptococcus pyogenes*.[57] This effect appears to be glucocorticoid dependent; administration of a glucocorticoid receptor antagonist eliminated the impact of stress on epidermis antimicrobial peptide production, and administration of exogenous glucocorticoid mimicked the effects of stress on antimicrobial production.[57]

Wound Hypoxia

Oxygen homeostasis is critical to all phases of wound healing. Damage created to blood vessels during wounding decreases oxygen availability. Simultaneously, neutrophils' oxidative burst increases oxygen demand at the wound site. Restraint stress can further promote wound hypoxia.[58] Compared with controls, restraint-stressed mice had higher levels of inducible nitric oxide synthase levels, an indicator of wound hypoxia at the wound site.[58] Furthermore, hyperbaric oxygen therapy normalized inducible nitric oxide synthase levels and attenuated stress-induced impairments in wound healing.[58]

BEHAVIORAL MECHANISMS LINKING STRESS AND WOUND HEALING

In addition to directly modulating physiologic responses to skin damage, stress can also indirectly influence wound repair by promoting the adoption of health-damaging behaviors. Individuals who experience greater levels of stress are more likely to increase their alcohol and tobacco use, decrease their participation in physical activity, experience sleep disturbances, and make poorer diet choices than individuals reporting less distress.[59,60] These negative health behavior practices can then compound the detrimental impact of stress on physiologic healing processes.[2]

Heavy alcohol use has been associated with delays in cell migration and collagen deposition at the wound site, which in turn can impede the healing process.[61] Smoking has also been related to slowed healing of naturally occurring and surgical wounds.[62] Sleep disruption delays skin barrier recovery after tape stripping and diminishes growth hormone production.[21,63] Lack of regular physical activity can slow the rate of wound healing.[36] Furthermore, deficient intake of glucose, polyunsaturated proteins, and certain vitamins can impede the healing process.[64–66]

SUMMARY

The goal of this review is to present clinical and experimental models of the impact of stress on wound repair. Converging and replicated evidence from experimental and clinical models of wound healing indicates that psychological stress leads to clinically relevant delays in wound healing. New mechanistic data suggest ways to elucidate the multiple physiologic pathways by which stress alters wound repair processes. Translational work should focus on identifying conditions in which behavioral and pharmacologic treatments are the most effective and on developing new treatments able to attenuate stress-induced delays in wound healing.

REFERENCES

1. Walburn J, Vedhara K, Hankins M, et al. Psychological stress and wound healing in humans: a systematic review and meta-analysis. J Psychosom Res 2009;67(3): 253–71.
2. Kiecolt-Glaser JK, Page GG, Marucha PT, et al. Psychological influences on surgical recovery: perspectives from psychoneuroimmunology. Am Psychol 1998;53:1209–18.
3. Rosenberger PH, Jokl P, Ickovics J. Psychosocial factors and surgical outcomes: an evidence-based literature review. J Am Acad Orthop Surg 2006;14(7): 397–405.
4. Boeke S, Duivenvoorden HJ, Verhage F, et al. Prediction of postoperative pain and duration of hospitalization using two anxiety measures. Pain 1991;45(3): 293–7.
5. Scheier MF, Matthews KA, Owens JF, et al. Optimism and rehospitalization after coronary artery bypass graft surgery. Arch Intern Med 1999;159:829–35.
6. Doering LV, Moser DK, Lemankiewicz W, et al. Depression, healing, and recovery from coronary artery bypass surgery. Am J Crit Care 2005;14(4):316–24.
7. Cole-King A, Harding KG. Psychological factors and delayed healing in chronic wounds. Psychosom Med 2001;63:216–20.
8. Gouin JP, Hantsoo L, Kiecolt-Glaser JK. Immune dysregulation and chronic stress among older adults: a review. Neuroimmunomodulation 2008;15(4–6):251–9.
9. Kiecolt-Glaser JK, Marucha PT, Malarkey WB, et al. Slowing of wound healing by psychological stress. Lancet 1995;346:1194–6.
10. Ebrecht M, Hextall J, Kirtley LG, et al. Perceived stress and cortisol levels predict speed of wound heating in healthy male adults. Psychoneuroendocrinology 2004; 29(6):798–809.
11. McGuire L, Heffner K, Glaser R, et al. Pain and wound healing in surgical patients. Ann Behav Med 2006;31(2):165–72.
12. Graham JE, Robles TF, Kiecolt-Glaser JK, et al. Hostility and pain are related to inflammation in older adults. Brain Behav Immun 2006;20(4):389–400.
13. Padgett DA, Marucha PT, Sheridan JF. Restraint stress slows cutaneous wound healing in mice. Brain Behav Immun 1998;12:64–73.
14. French SS, Matt KS, Moore MC. The effects of stress on wound healing in male tree lizards (Urosaurus ornatus). Gen Comp Endocrinol 2006;145(2):128–32.
15. Martin LB 2nd, Glasper ER, Nelson RJ, et al. Prolonged separation delays wound healing in monogamous California mice, Peromyscus californicus, but not in polygynous white-footed mice, P. leucopus. Physiol Behav 2006;87(5):837–41.

16. Marucha PT, Kiecolt-Glaser JK, Favagehi M. Mucosal wound healing is impaired by examination stress. Psychosom Med 1998;60:362–5.
17. Bosch JA, Engeland CG, Cacioppo JT, et al. Depressive symptoms predict mucosal wound healing. Psychosom Med 2007;69(7):597–605.
18. Kiecolt-Glaser JK, Loving TJ, Stowell JR, et al. Hostile marital interactions, proinflammatory cytokine production, and wound healing. Arch Gen Psychiatry 2005; 62:1377–84.
19. Gouin JP, Carter CS, Pournajafi-Nazarloo H, et al. Marital behavior, oxytocin, vasopressin, and wound healing. Psychoneuroendocrinology 2010;35(7):1082–90.
20. Gouin JP, Kiecolt-Glaser JK, Malarkey WB, et al. The influence of anger expression on wound healing. Brain Behav Immun 2008;22(5):699–708.
21. Altemus M, Rao B, Dhabhar FS, et al. Stress-induced changes in skin barrier function in healthy women. J Invest Dermatol 2001;117:309–17.
22. Dickerson SS, Kemeny ME. Acute stressors and cortisol responses: a theoretical integration and synthesis of laboratory research. Psychol Bull 2004;130(3):355–91.
23. Kirschbaum C, Pirke KM, Hellhammer DH. The "Trier social stress test"—a tool for investigating psychobiological stress responses in a laboratory setting. Neuropsychobiology 1993;28:76–81.
24. Robles TF. Stress, social support, and delayed skin barrier recovery. Psychosom Med 2007;69(8):807–15.
25. Robles TF, Brooks KP, Pressman SD. Trait positive affect buffers the effects of acute stress on skin barrier recovery. Health Psychol 2009;28(3):373–8.
26. Garg A, Chren MM, Sands LP, et al. Psychological stress perturbs epidermal permeability barrier homeostasis: implications for the pathogenesis of stress-associated skin disorders. Arch Dermatol 2000;137:53–9.
27. Muizzuddin N, Matsui MS, Marenus KD, et al. Impact of stress of marital dissolution on skin barrier recovery: tape stripping and measurement of trans-epidermal water loss (TEWL). Skin Res Technol 2003;9:34–8.
28. Denda M, Tsuchiya T, Hosoi J, et al. Immobilization-induced and crowded environment-induced stress delay barrier recovery in murine skin. Br J Dermatol 1998;138:780–5.
29. Denda M, Tsuchiya T, Elias PM, et al. Stress alters cutaneous permeability barrier homeostasis. Am J Physiol Regul Integr Comp Physiol 2000;278:R367–72.
30. Johnston M, Vogele C. Benefits of psychological preparation for surgery: a meta-analysis. Ann Behav Med 1993;15:245–56.
31. Montgomery GH, David D, Winkel G, et al. The effectiveness of adjunctive hypnosis with surgical patients: a meta-analysis. Anesth Analg 2002;94(6): 1639–45, [table of contents].
32. Esterling BA, L'Abate L, Murray EJ, et al. Empirical foundations for writing in prevention and psychotherapy: mental and physical health outcomes. Clin Psychol Rev 1999;19(1):79–96.
33. Weinman J, Ebrecht M, Scott S, et al. Enhanced wound healing after emotional disclosure intervention. Br J Health Psychol 2008;13(Pt 1):95–102.
34. Emery CF, Blumenthal JA. Effects of physical exercise on psychological and cognitive functioning of older adults. Ann Behav Med 1991;13:99–107.
35. Emery CF, Kiecolt-Glaser JK, Glaser R, et al. Exercise accelerates wound healing among healthy older adults: a preliminary investigation. J Gerontol A Biol Sci Med Sci 2005;60(11):1432–6.
36. Keylock KT, Vieira VJ, Wallig MA, et al. Exercise accelerates cutaneous wound healing and decreases wound inflammation in aged mice. Am J Physiol Regul Integr Comp Physiol 2008;294(1):R179–84.

37. House JS, Landis KR, Umberson D. Social relationships and health. Science 1988;241:540–5.
38. Glasper ER, Devries AC. Social structure influences effects of pair-housing on wound healing. Brain Behav Immun 2005;19(1):61–8.
39. Detillion CE, Craft TK, Glasper ER, et al. Social facilitation of wound healing. Psychoneuroendocrinology 2004;29(8):1004–11.
40. Rossi A, Barraco A, Donda P. Fluoxetine: a review on evidence based medicine. Ann Gen Hosp Psychiatry 2004;3(1):2.
41. Farahani RM, Sadr K, Rad JS, et al. Fluoxetine enhances cutaneous wound healing in chronically stressed Wistar rats. Adv Skin Wound Care 2007;20(3):157–65.
42. Hubner G, Brauchle M, Smola H, et al. Differential regulation of pro-inflammatory cytokines during wound healing in normal glucocorticoid-treated mice. Cytokine 1996;8(7):548–56.
43. Werner S, Grose R. Regulation of wound healing by growth factors and cytokines. Physiol Rev 2003;83(3):835–70.
44. Gallucci RM, Simeonova PP, Matheson JM, et al. Impaired cutaneous wound healing in interleukin-6-deficient and immunosuppressed mice. FASEB J 2000; 14:2525–31.
45. Padgett DA, Glaser R. How stress influences the immune response. Trends Immunol 2003;24(8):444–8.
46. Glaser R, Kiecolt-Glaser JK. Stress-induced immune dysfunction: implications for health. Nat Rev Immunol 2005;5:243–51.
47. Eijkelkamp N, Engeland CG, Gajendrareddy PK, et al. Restraint stress impairs early wound healing in mice via alpha-adrenergic but not beta-adrenergic receptors. Brain Behav Immun 2007;21(4):409–12.
48. Romana-Souza B, Otranto M, Vieira AM, et al. Rotational stress-induced increase in epinephrine levels delays cutaneous wound healing in mice. Brain Behav Immun 2010;24(3):427–37.
49. Sivamani RK, Pullar CE, Manabat-Hidalgo CG, et al. Stress-mediated increases in systemic and local epinephrine impair skin wound healing: potential new indication for beta blockers. PLoS Med 2009;6(1):e12.
50. Vitalo A, Fricchione J, Casali M, et al. Nest making and oxytocin comparably promote wound healing in isolation reared rats. PLoS One 2009;4(5):e5523.
51. Glaser R, Kiecolt-Glaser JK, Marucha PT, et al. Stress-related changes in proinflammatory cytokine production in wounds. Arch Gen Psychiatry 1999; 56:450–6.
52. Broadbent E, Petrie KJ, Alley PG, et al. Psychological stress impairs early wound repair following surgery. Psychosom Med 2003;65(5):865–9.
53. Mercado AM, Padgett DA, Sheridan JF, et al. Altered kinetics of IL-1 alpha, IL-1 beta, and KGF-1 gene expression in early wounds of restrained mice. Brain Behav Immun 2002;16(2):150–62.
54. Head CC, Farrow MJ, Sheridan JF, et al. Androstenediol reduces the anti-inflammatory effects of restraint stress during wound healing. Brain Behav Immun 2006; 20(6):590–6.
55. Yang EV, Bane CM, MacCallum RC, et al. Stress-related modulation of matrix metalloproteinase expression. J Neuroimmunol 2002;133(1–2):144–50.
56. Rojas I, Padgett DA, Sheridan JF, et al. Stress-induced susceptibility to bacterial infection during cutaneous wound healing. Brain Behav Immun 2002;16:74–84.
57. Aberg KM, Radek KA, Choi EH, et al. Psychological stress downregulates epidermal antimicrobial peptide expression and increases severity of cutaneous infections in mice. J Clin Invest 2007;117(11):3339–49.

58. Gajendrareddy PK, Sen CK, Horan MP, et al. Hyperbaric oxygen therapy ameliorates stress-impaired dermal wound healing. Brain Behav Immun 2005;19(3): 217–22.

59. Steptoe A, Wardle J, Pollard TM, et al. Stress, social support and health-related behavior: a study of smoking, alcohol consumption and physical exercise. J Psychosom Res 1996;41:171–80.

60. Vitaliano PP, Scanlan JM, Zhang J, et al. A path model of chronic stress, the metabolic syndrome, and coronary heart disease. Psychosom Med 2002;64:418–35.

61. Benveniste K, Thut P. The effect of chronic alcoholism on wound healing. Proc Soc Exp Biol Med 1981;166:568–75.

62. Silverstein P. Smoking and wound healing. Am J Med 1992;93:22S–4S.

63. Veldhuis JD, Iranmanesch A. Physiological regulation of the human growth hormone (GH)-insulin-like growth factor type I (IGF-I) axis: predominant impact of age, obesity, gonadal function, and sleep. Sleep 1996;19:S221–4.

64. Russell L. The importance of patients' nutritional status in wound healing. Br J Nurs 2001;10(6 Suppl):S42, S44–9.

65. Posthauer ME. The role of nutrition in wound care. Adv Skin Wound Care 2006; 19(1):43–52 [quiz: 53–4].

66. McDaniel JC, Belury M, Ahijevych K, et al. Omega-3 fatty acids effect on wound healing. Wound Repair Regen 2008;16(3):337–45.

Neuroendocrine Effects of Stress on Immunity in the Elderly: Implications for Inflammatory Disease

Kathi L. Heffner, PhD

KEYWORDS

- Stress • HPA axis • Inflammation • Inflammatory disease
- Aging • Older adults

Aging is accompanied by immunosenescence, a gradual and natural change in immune system structure and function. Many of these changes lead to substantial immune dysregulation, leaving older adults at increased risk for infection, compromised wound healing, and poor oral health. Immunosenescence is also implicated in chronic, low-level inflammation that is linked to a host of chronic, age-related diseases, including rheumatoid arthritis, atherosclerosis, osteoporosis, and type-2 diabetes.[1–3] The relative balance of the production of inflammatory mediators by subsets of T-helper (Th) cells, namely Th1 and Th2 cells, also shifts with aging and has consequences for immunity and health in the elderly.[4] Psychological stress has similar costs: chronic stress, such as ongoing interpersonal strain or caregiving for a spouse with dementia, has many of the same dysregulating effects on inflammatory processes as seen with aging.[5] Thus, there may be potentially additive or synergistic effects of immunosenescence and stress on immune and inflammatory dysregulation in older adults, further increasing disease risk.

The physiologic stress response is a function of the dynamic interplay among the nervous, endocrine, and immune systems, and is intended to promote adaptation and homeostasis in the face of environmental challenges (a violent aggressor) or physical stressors (tissue injury or infection). Psychological stressors, such as worry, anxiety, and perceived lack of control, also activate stress systems to support adaptation by the organism. When chronically or repeatedly activated, however, the products of these systems can damage tissues and contribute to disease development.[6]

This work was supported by National Institute on Aging grant R24 AG031089–01.
The author has nothing to disclose.
Department of Psychiatry, The Rochester Center for Mind-Body Research, University of Rochester Medical Center, 300 Crittenden Boulevard, Box PSYCH-BPSM, Rochester, NY 14642, USA
E-mail address: Kathi_Heffner@urmc.rochester.edu

For older adults, physiologic activation in response to stressors is transposed upon age-related dysregulation of stress-response systems. Neuroendocrine activation is the primary stimulus for fight–flight responses, originating in the hypothalamus and resulting in secretion of the so-called stress hormones by the adrenal glands. Adrenal hormones released in response to stress, including glucocorticoids, dehydroepian-drosterone (DHEA), and the catecholamines, epinephrine (EP), and norepinephrine (NE), can each independently modulate immune function. Importantly, neuroendo-crine function, like immune function, is altered with both aging and chronic stress.[7,8] Accordingly, aging and stress-related neuroendocrine dysregulation may combine to further disrupt immune function, increasing risk for or exacerbating inflammatory disease in older adults. This article highlights evidence for the impact of age and stress on adrenal stress hormone regulation of inflammatory processes that may substan-tially increase risk for inflammatory disease at older ages.

AGING, STRESS, AND INFLAMMATORY PROCESSES

Immunosenescence is characterized by two, interrelated changes in inflammatory activity that can place older adults at risk for chronic, inflammatory diseases. The first relates to chronic activation of innate, inflammatory responses, marked by increasing levels and impaired synthesis of proinflammatory cytokines, especially interleukin (IL)-6.[9] Indeed, IL-6 is a potent predictor of mortality in older adults,[10,11] and IL-6 and other proinflammatory mediators have been implicated in the development of a host of inflammatory diseases, including cardiovascular disease, type 2 diabetes, osteoporosis, and arthritis.[12–14]

Age-related changes in adaptive or acquired cell-mediated immunity also occur and are accompanied by changes in Th1 and Th2 effector cell activity. Th1 cells primarily secrete IL-2, interferon gamma (IFN-γ), and tumor necrosis factor beta (TNF-β), required for cell-mediated inflammatory reactions that can efficiently eliminate intracellular path-ogens. Th2 cells primarily secrete IL-4, IL-5, IL-10, and IL-13, required for humoral immu-nity. IL-4 and IL-10 stimulate B cells to produce antigen and immunoglobulin (Ig) switching to IgE, as well as mast cell and eosinophil growth and activation.[15,16]

Th1 and Th2 cytokines are mutually inhibitory and, ideally, maintain a homeostatic equilibrium between cell-mediated and humoral responses.[17,18] Aging, however, is asso-ciated with a decline in this equilibrium. Th1 cytokine secretion declines with advancing age, particularly the expression of IL-2,[19] and there is a shift toward a Th2 anti-inflamma-tory response, marked by increases in IL-10 secretion and expression.[20,21] Such shifts have proposed links to increased risk for or exacerbation of atopic allergy, allergic rhinitis, asthma, autoimmunity, and chronic infection in susceptible individuals.[17,22–24]

Notably, chronic stress, like age, is associated with increases in circulating levels of proinflammatory cytokines,[4,12,25,26] as well as a shift toward Th2 responses.[17,18,21] Age and chronic stress are also each associated with changes in adrenal stress hormone function, which, in light of substantial hormonal modulation of inflammatory activity, may play a prominent role in exacerbating effects of stress on inflammation, Th1 to Th2 shift, and relevant disease risk in older adults. Changes in these relevant aspects of immunologic and endocrinological function are depicted in **Fig. 1**.

THE NEUROENDOCRINE STRESS RESPONSE AND MODULATION OF IMMUNITY: AGE EFFECTS

The aging and remodeling of the endocrine system—endocrinosenescence—is closely related to immunosenescence, due to the immunomodulating properties of endocrine hormones.[27] Endocrine dysregulation affects the course and consequences of activation

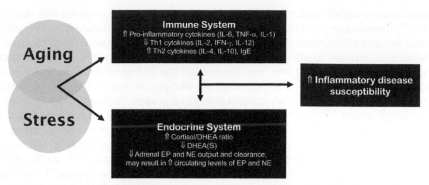

Fig. 1. Aging and stress each impact endocrine and immune function, affecting regulation of inflammatory mediators and adrenal stress hormones. Stress-related dysregulation of these systems may combine with age-related dysregulation to render older adults particularly vulnerable to inflammatory disease. DHEA(S), dehydroepiandrosterone (DHEA) and DHEA sulfate.

of the hypothalamic-pituitary-adrenal (HPA) axis and the sympathetic-adrenal-medullary (SAM) axis, which together coordinate physiologic responses to stress.

Comprehensive reviews of the physiologic stress response are available.[28,29] Briefly, in response to both physical and psychological stressors, and integrating input from processing centers, including the amygdala, prefrontal cortex, and hippocampus, the hypothalamus releases corticotropin-releasing hormone (CRH) from the paraventricular nucleus. CRH stimulates the pituitary gland to release adrenocorticotropic hormone (ACTH). From the brain, ACTH enters circulation and ultimately stimulates the cortex of the adrenal glands to produce glucocorticoids, of which cortisol is the primary stress hormone secreted in humans. Other androgens can be released as well, including DHEA, an endogenous hormone that regulates activities of cortisol, although its physiologic significance and role in disease are not well understood.[30,31] In parallel, owing to hypothalamic sympathetic innervation of the adrenal gland's medulla, sympathetic activation results in release of catecholamines into circulation, including EP and NE. Together, cortisol and EP upregulate glucose metabolism and cardiovascular activity to support fight or flight. Cortisol also suppresses aspects of immune activity during stress, whereas DHEA may serve to moderate these immunosuppressive affects, as DHEA is shown to antagonize effects of glucocorticoids.

Thus, the HPA axis is a dynamic, regulatory system that supports life-sustaining adjustments aimed at maintaining homeostasis and is, thus, one of the most important allostatic or adaptive systems.[32] Aging, however, is associated with changes in HPA axis morphology and function that affect cortisol, DHEA, and catecholamine regulation in response to stress. These HPA changes, in turn, affect regulation of inflammatory processes.

Cortisol

Age-related changes

Secretion of glucocorticoids by the HPA axis occurs through spontaneous, pulsatile, circadian fluctuations, as well as in response to stress, and has widespread affects on immune function under both basal and stressful conditions. Cortisol secretion is maintained with advancing age. Evidence from animal and human studies suggests that glucocorticoid levels remain constant throughout adulthood[32,33] and may even increase[7,34,35]; although observed diurnal increases may be more evident among distressed older adults[36] or individuals with impairments in physical functioning.[37] Other studies indicate higher nocturnal levels of cortisol among older compared with younger adults,[32,38] resulting in greater overall cortisol circulation across the diurnal cycle. Further, cortisol remains elevated relative to age-related declines in other adrenal hormones.[39]

Aging also appears to affect glucocorticoid output in response to HPA activation, although evidence is mixed and may depend on the source of activation as well as subject characteristics. In pharmacologic challenge studies, CRH administration increases circulating and salivary cortisol levels to a greater degree in older compared with younger adults.[40–42] Age is also associated with a reduced suppression of cortisol secretion by dexamethasone, though age-related effects may be stronger in women.[40] Psychological challenge studies show greater inconsistency, with some studies supporting age-related increases in cortisol response,[43,44] while others show no age differences[41,45] or reduced responsiveness in older adults.[46] There are apparent gender differences, as well as other factors that modify the influence of age on cortisol response, such as fitness level.[47] In a recent meta-analysis,[42] age had stronger effects on cortisol responses to pharmacologic and psychosocial challenges in women compared with men. However, older men overall show larger cortisol responses to psychological stress compared with older women,[44,48] a gender effect consistently observed across the age range.[49] Mixed findings from stress reactivity studies comparing men versus women, and older and younger adults, may be due to a host of factors. For example, there is evidence that sex steroids, which of course vary by age and gender, modulate HPA reactivity.[49] Further, different kinds of stressors (eg, interpersonal vs cognitive) and other psychosocial factors (eg, social environment) modulate cortisol reactivity differently in men versus women,[50] and older versus younger adults.[51] Thus, the nature of the stressor used in research must be considered when interpreting age and gender differences.

Major contributors to age-related changes in cortisol regulation and responses to stress include age-related impairments in negative feedback sensitivity of the HPA axis to cortisol,[40,52] increased adrenal sensitivity to ACTH,[53] and the decline of adrenal hormones, such as DHEA, that regulate cortisol production.[8] Glucocorticoids are key regulators of inflammatory responses during and following stress, and contribute to stress-related shifts toward Th2 responses.[16] Thus, age-related dysregulation of cortisol secretion may substantially impact regulation of inflammatory responses during a stress response, thereby increasing older adults' risk for inflammatory disease.

Regulation of proinflammatory cytokines

Glucocorticoids have strong anti-inflammatory effects, primarily mediated through their interaction with glucocorticoid receptors (GR) maintained in the cytoplasm of immune cells. GR activation inhibits inflammatory cytokine production by blocking the activation of transcription factors, such as NF-κB, that are responsible for cytokine gene expression.

The functional effects of glucocorticoids, however, depend on the sensitivity of target tissues to the hormones. For example, as noted above, aging reduces negative feedback sensitivity of the HPA axis, characterized by reduced glucocorticoid inhibition of CRH and ACTH secretion.[41,52] Stress and aging modulate glucocorticoid sensitivity in the immune system as well. Evidence suggests that glucocorticoid sensitivity of cytokine-producing immune cells is rapidly increased by physical stressors,[54] as well as acute psychological stressors,[45] resulting in substantial anti-inflammatory effects of glucocorticoids. Glucocorticoid sensitivity appears to be retained[55] or even increased at older ages.[45] On the contrary, more chronically stressful and distressing circumstances, such as low socioeconomic status in early life,[56] caring for a child with cancer,[57] or caregiving for a spouse with dementia,[36] are associated with resistance to anti-inflammatory effects of glucocorticoids. Further, glucocorticoid inhibition of IL-6 production was lower in older men compared with younger men following psychological stress-induced HPA activation,[58] and treatment with testosterone diminished the age-related reduction in stress-induced glucocorticoid resistance. Finally, glucocorticoid resistance in certain inflammatory diseases, such as steroid-resistant asthma, rheumatoid arthritis, and inflammatory bowel disease, is well-documented.[59,60]

Glucocorticoid resistance can develop through various pathways, including genetic susceptibility, down-regulation of glucocorticoid receptors and alterations in the expression of transcription factors necessary for glucocorticoid signaling.[61,62] These pathways are regulated by both glucocorticoids and proinflammatory cytokines.[62] For example, glucocorticoids can downregulate glucocorticoid receptor expression,[63] and proinflammatory cytokines can activate transcription pathways that inhibit glucocorticoid receptor signaling.[64] Thus, combined influences of age and stress on increases in proinflammatory cytokine production and cortisol may further exacerbate alterations in glucocorticoid sensitivity and consequent inflammation in older adults.

Regulation of Th1 and Th2 responses
Glucocorticoids have strong effects on Th1 and Th2 responses. Cortisol can inhibit production of IL-12,[17] a major inducer of Th1 responses. Glucocorticoids also suppress Th1 cytokines directly, including production of IFN-γ and IL-2, leaving intact or augmenting production of Th2 cytokines, including IL-4 and IL-10.[65,66] As a result, glucocorticoids can enhance Th2 functions, such as production of IgE. In prior clinical studies, stress was associated with elevated IgE.[67,68] Kiecolt-Glaser and colleagues[69] (including the author) recently demonstrated the ability of stress and anxiety to enhance allergen-specific IgE responses. Further, altered HPA responsiveness is observed in inflammatory diseases.[23,70] Thus, altered stress responsiveness of the HPA axis with advancing age may contribute to dysregulation of Th1 and Th2 cytokine production and increase older adults' risk for Th1 and Th2-mediated inflammatory disease.

In addition, activation and termination of an immune response depends on complex interactions between the innate and adaptive arms of immunity, specifically, interactions of antigen presenting cells (APCs), and T cells, respectively. As noted, IL-12 is the primary stimulator of TH1 responses. IL-12 is produced by APCs, including monocytes, macrophages, and dendritic cells. These cells also secrete the anti-inflammatory cytokine IL-10. Studies show increases in both IL-12 and IL-10 with aging, suggesting a possible compensatory process.[20] There is also evidence for age-related impairment of communication between APCs and T cells.[20] The role of stress hormones in changes in APC cell-to-T cell communication as a function of age or stress remains to be characterized.

DHEA

Age-related changes
DHEA and its inactive precursor, DHEA sulfate (DHEAS), are the most abundant adrenal steroid hormones in circulation in humans,[71] and their steady decline with advancing age is a well-recognized pattern.[30] DHEA(S) peak during the third decade of life and by the end of the eighth decade are at 10% to 30% of peak levels.[32,72,73] The age-related decline is believed to be due primarily to the morphologic changes of the adrenal cortex, particularly the reduction in size of the zona reticularis,[74,75] the exclusive source of DHEA. The extent of age-related decline in DHEA(S), however, shows marked interindividual variability.[76] There may also be gender differences. In two studies, women showed less decline relative to men[77,78]; although Mazat and colleagues[79] found greater decline in women.

Like cortisol, DHEA is secreted by the adrenal cortex in response to CRH and ACTH stimulation,[33] and there is evidence that both pharmacologic challenges and psychological stressors provoke increases in circulating and salivary levels of DHEA(S) in humans[80,81] and nonhuman primates.[82] Less is known about how stress-responsivity of DHEA(S) is affected by age, but older individuals show reduced DHEA secretion in response to ACTH stimulation compared with younger individuals.[83] Importantly, DHEA and cortisol have opposing effects on immune function,[84] and the cortisol/DHEA ratio increases with age. Thus, the cortisol/DHEA ratio may provide more information about neuroendocrine-immune interactions that compromise health at older ages.[7,85]

Regulation of inflammatory processes

DHEA has a direct effect on cytokine-producing monocytes and lymphocytes, and evidence suggests its potential role in reducing the inflammatory affects of immunosenescence. DHEA diminished IL-6 secretion by lymphoid cells of aged mice[86] and murine macrophages stimulated with lipopolysaccharide (LPS).[87] DHEA was shown to increase Th1 cytokines[86,88,89] and inhibit in vitro IL-6 secretion in a study of postmenopausal women.[90]

DHEA may also affect inflammatory cytokine production indirectly through its suppressive effects on cortisol production.[8] Animal models of trauma show that supplementation with DHEA can attenuate the trauma-related rise in corticosterone and enhance T cell secretion of IL-2, IL-3 and IFN-γ, thereby restoring splenocyte proliferation that is typically depressed following traumatic injury.[88] As noted, the ratio of cortisol to DHEA increases with age; thus, the decline in DHEA and resulting glucocorticoid excess together may impact on inflammatory function under basal conditions and in response to stress.

In addition, downstream products of DHEA synthesis may be primarily responsible for attenuation of age-related inflammatory dysregulation, as others have shown sex steroids and other androgens for which DHEA is a precursor to modulate inflammatory cytokine production.[91] For example, age-related immunosuppression was associated with a Th1 (IFN-γ) to Th2 (IL-4) shift in burn-injured mice,[92] and a significantly greater increase in IL-6.[93] In both cases, the effect of age on cytokine production was reduced with estrogen treatment. Indeed, evidence has accumulated that sex steroids are key inflammatory regulators.[94]

Evidence regarding the suppressive versus enhancing effects of DHEA on proinflammatory cytokine production is equivocal, however. IL-6 production by human monocytes stimulated by LPS was enhanced by DHEA.[95] T-cells from DHEA-treated older men, when stimulated with nonspecific mitogen, also showed enhanced IL-6 production, but IL-2 production was also improved,[96] suggesting an enhanced Th1 response. In contrast, DHEA supplementation had little influence on mitogen-stimulated IL-6 production in a study of postmenopausal women,[97] although other immune effects of DHEA were found, including enhancement of natural killer cell cytotoxicity. It has been suggested that the mixed findings in human studies may be due to inconsistent DHEA exposure (for example, longer-term in vivo administration vs short-term administration in vitro[98]) and supplementation dosage.[8] In spite of mixed findings, DHEA supplementation continues to be regarded as a promising approach to reduce age-associated risks for inflammatory diseases.[8,98,99]

Sympathoadrenal Hormones

Age-related changes

Compared to the other adrenal stress hormones, much less is known about aging effects on the SAM axis regulation of inflammatory processes. The sympathetic nervous system (SNS) shows changes with age, with increased overall tonic activity at rest, primarily indexed by NE output at neuroeffector junctions (that is, NE in its neuro-transmitter form) using tracer technologies.[100,101] Enhanced SNS activity, however, is seen in some tissue regions but not others.[102–104] Higher basal circulating levels of NE have also been observed in older compared with younger men.[100,105] In contrast, EP output by the adrenal medulla under resting conditions was shown to decline with age,[106] whereas others had reported a slight decline or no change in circulating levels of EP with aging.[107,108] However, age-related reductions in EP clearance from circulation can obscure interpretations about EP output by the adrenal medulla when measuring circulating catecholamine levels.[103]

The same interpretation constraints may also contribute to mixed findings regarding age effects on SAM responses to stress. Adrenal catecholamine output in response to stress also appears to decline with age.[103,106] Again, however, age-related declines in catecholamine clearance may have led to the larger increases in circulating levels of NE observed in older adults relative to younger adults following physical and psychological stressors.[109,110] Others have not found age to affect circulating NE in response to stress.[100,111] In addition, NE spillover from neuroeffector junctions into circulation increases with age[103]; thus it is unclear whether circulating levels of NE are more a function of spillover or age-related changes in NE output by the adrenal medulla.

In sum, relatively little is known about the effects of age on sympathoadrenal activity during stress, but evidence suggests there may be age-related differences in adrenal output and clearance of catecholamines. The health implications of these age-related changes remain to be determined.

Regulation of inflammatory processes

The SNS has immunomodulating properties,[112–114] but less is known about regulation of inflammatory cytokines by in vivo actions of catecholamines secreted by the adrenal medulla during stress. However, EP and cortisol appear to combine to regulate inflammatory cytokine production. For example, under basal conditions, EP was recently shown to enhance LPS-induced production of the anti-inflammatory cytokine IL-10 by monocytes, while inhibiting proinflammatory TNF-α and IL-12[22]; basal cortisol levels did not regulate production of these cytokines ex vivo. In contrast, in vitro studies indicate that both physiologic stress levels of glucocorticoids and EP inhibit production of IL-12, the potent stimulator of Th1 responses.[66] Further, EP and corticosteroids in vitro decrease Th1 cytokine production and increase Th2 cytokine production to a significantly greater degree compared with either adrenal hormone alone.[115] It is unclear how age-related changes in HPA function affect these regulatory pathways.

Taken together, adrenally secreted catecholamines, specifically EP, play a role in both innate proinflammatory cytokine regulation, as well as adaptive Th responses, and may act in concert with cortisol during stress to modulate cytokine activity. Indeed, both hyporesponsiveness of the HPA axis and hyperresponsiveness of the SAM axis to psychological stress have been observed in patients with atopic dermatitis, a chronic inflammatory disease primarily mediated by Th2 inflammatory responses,[70] further underscoring coregulatory contributions of these stress hormones. The age-related decline in EP output might be expected to affect inflammatory cytokine regulation and subsequent disease susceptibility; alternatively, age-related reductions in EP clearance may serve a compensatory function.

SUMMARY

Advances in our understanding of neuroendocrine–immune interactions suggest that endocrinosenescence and immunosenescence are tightly linked through hormones and inflammatory cytokines.[116] Evidence further suggests that some of the biologic sequelae of stress mimic those observed in human aging, and include increased production of proinflammatory cytokines and an impairment of the Th1-Th2 balance. Age-related changes in the HPA axis and in regulatory control of inflammatory processes by stress hormones render older adults vulnerable to inflammatory disease. Transposing stress onto age-related changes in endocrine and inflammatory function likely exacerbates these disease risks. Indeed, greater immunosuppressive effects of stress, such as antibody response to vaccination, have been observed in older adults compared with younger adults.[117]

There remain important questions about the potential additive or synergistic affects of stress and biologic aging that may increase older adults' risk for inflammatory disease. First, although this article highlights the regulatory control of stress hormones on inflammatory processes, inflammatory cytokines regulate the HPA axis as well.[118] Therefore, elucidation of age effects on this regulatory pathway is needed. Further, a systems-level approach is necessary to fully understand the pathophysiology of age-related changes in immunity,[13,116] and its contribution to disease development. A full model of the inflammatory disease implications of stress and aging must account for the mutual regulation of the endocrine and immune systems. Finally, it has become increasingly clear that immunosenescence is a function of lifetime exposure to pathogens.[119] Models of stress and health suggest that lifetime exposure to stress also contributes to biologic aging.[120,121] Thus, developmental changes in the interplay of stress hormones and inflammatory processes must be considered to fully understand the implications of neuroendocrine stress responses for inflammatory disease risk in the elderly.

REFERENCES

1. Franceschi C, Bonafe M, Valensin S, et al. Inflamm-aging. An evolutionary perspective on immunosenescence. Ann N Y Acad Sci 2000;908:244–54.
2. Kiecolt-Glaser JK, Preacher KJ, MacCallum RC, et al. Chronic stress and age-related increases in the proinflammatory cytokine IL-6. Proc Natl Acad Sci U S A 2003;100:9090–5.
3. Papanicolaou DA, Wilder RL, Manolagas SC, et al. The pathophysiologic roles of interleukin-6 in human disease. Ann Intern Med 1998;128:127–37.
4. Elenkov IJ, Iezzoni DG, Daly A, et al. Cytokine dysregulation, inflammation and well-being. Neuroimmunomodulation 2005;12:255–69.
5. Hawkley LC, Cacioppo JT. Stress and the aging immune system. Brain Behav Immun 2004;18:114–9.
6. McEwen BS. Central effects of stress hormones in health and disease: understanding the protective and damaging effects of stress and stress mediators. Eur J Pharmacol 2008;583:174–85.
7. Bauer ME. Stress, glucocorticoids and ageing of the immune system. Stress 2005;8:69–83.
8. Butcher SK, Lord JM, Butcher SK, et al. Stress responses and innate immunity: aging as a contributory factor. Aging Cell 2004;3:151–60.
9. Ershler WB, Keller ET. Age-associated increased interleukin-6 gene expression, late-life diseases, and frailty. Annu Rev Med 2000;51:245–70.
10. Gruenewald TL, Seeman TE, Ryff CD, et al. Combinations of biomarkers predictive of later life mortality. Proc Natl Acad Sci U S A 2006;103:14158–63.
11. Harris TB, Ferrucci L, Tracy RP, et al. Associations of elevated interleukin-6 and C-reactive protein levels with mortality in the elderly. Am J Med 1999;106: 506–12.

12. Black PH. The inflammatory consequences of psychologic stress: relationship to insulin resistance, obesity, atherosclerosis and diabetes mellitus, type II. Med Hypotheses 2006;67:879–91.
13. Giunta S. Exploring the complex relations between inflammation and aging (inflamm-aging): anti-inflamm-aging remodelling of inflamm- aging, from robustness to frailty. Inflamm Res 2008;57:558–63.
14. van Leeuwen MA, Westra J, Limburg PC, et al. Clinical significance of interleukin-6 measurement in early rheumatoid arthritis: relation with laboratory and clinical variables and radiological progression in a three year prospective study. Ann Rheum Dis 1995;54:674–7.
15. Diehl S, Rincon M. The two faces of IL-6 on Th1/Th2 differentiation. Mol Immunol 2002;39:531–6.
16. Elenkov IJ. Neurohormonal-cytokine interactions: implications for inflammation, common human diseases and well-being. Neurochem Int 2008;52:40–51.
17. Elenkov IJ, Chrousos GP. Stress hormones, Th1/Th2 patterns, pro/anti-inflammatory cytokines and susceptibility to disease. Trends Endocrinol Metab 1999;10:359–68.
18. Marshall GD Jr, Agarwal SK, Lloyd C, et al. Cytokine dysregulation associated with exam stress in healthy medical students. Brain Behav Immun 1998;12:297–307.
19. Rink L, Cakman I, Kirchner H. Altered cytokine production in the elderly. Mech Ageing Dev 1998;102:199–209.
20. Castle SC. Clinical relevance of age-related immune dysfunction. Clin Infect Dis 2000;31:578–85.
21. Glaser R, MacCallum RC, Laskowski BF, et al. Evidence for a shift in the Th-1 to Th-2 cytokine response associated with chronic stress and aging. J Gerontol A Biol Sci Med Sci 2001;56:M477–82.
22. Elenkov IJ, Kvetnansky R, Hashiramoto A, et al. Low- versus high-baseline epinephrine output shapes opposite innate cytokine profiles: presence of Lewis- and Fischer-like neurohormonal immune phenotypes in humans? J Immunol 2008;181:1737–45.
23. Eskandari F, Webster JI, Sternberg EM. Neural immune pathways and their connection to inflammatory diseases. Arthritis Res Ther 2003;5:251–65.
24. Marshall GD. Neuroendocrine mechanisms of immune dysregulation: applications to allergy and asthma. Ann Allergy Asthma Immunol 2004;93:S11–7.
25. Brydon L, Walker C, Wawrzyniak A, et al. Synergistic effects of psychological and immune stressors on inflammatory cytokine and sickness responses in humans. Brain Behav Immun 2009;23:217–24.
26. Zhou D, Kusnecov AW, Shurin MR, et al. Exposure to physical and psychological stressors elevates plasma interleukin 6: relationship to the activation of hypothalamic-pituitary-adrenal axis. Endocrinology 1993;133:2523–30.
27. Straub RH, Gluck T, Cutolo M, et al. The adrenal steroid status in relation to inflammatory cytokines (interleukin-6 and tumour necrosis factor) in polymyalgia rheumatica. Rheumatology 2000;39:624–31.
28. Chrousos GP. Stress and disorders of the stress system. Nat Rev Endocrinol 2009;5:374–81.
29. Lovallo WR. Stress & health: biological and psychological interactions. 2nd edition. Thousand Oaks (CA): Sage; 2005.
30. Chahal HS, Drake WM. The endocrine system and ageing. J Pathol 2007;211:173–80.

31. Maninger N, Wolkowitz OM, Reus VI, et al. Neurobiological and neuropsychiatric effects of dehydroepiandrosterone (DHEA) and DHEA sulfate (DHEAS). Front Neuroendocrinol 2009;30:65–91.
32. Ferrari E, Cravello L, Muzzoni B, et al. Age-related changes of the hypothalamic-pituitary-adrenal axis: pathophysiological correlates. Eur J Endocrinol 2001;144: 319–29 European federation of endocrine societies.
33. Goncharova ND, Lapin BA. Effects of aging on hypothalamic-pituitary-adrenal system function in non-human primates. Mech Ageing Dev 2002;123:1191–201.
34. Born J, Ditschuneit I, Schreiber M, et al. Effects of age and gender on pituitary-adrenocortical responsiveness in humans. Eur J Endocrinol 1995;132:705–11 European federation of endocrine societies.
35. Seeman TE, Singer B, Wilkinson CW, et al. Gender differences in age-related changes in HPA axis reactivity. Psychoneuroendocrinology 2001;26:225–40.
36. Bauer ME, Vedhara K, Perks P, et al. Chronic stress in caregivers of dementia patients is associated with reduced lymphocyte sensitivity to glucocorticoids. J Neuroimmunol 2000;103:84–92.
37. Kumari M, Badrick E, Sacker A, et al. Identifying patterns in cortisol secretion in an older population. Findings from the Whitehall II study. Psychoneuroendocrinology 2010;35(7):1091–9.
38. Van Cauter E, Leproult R, Kupfer DJ. Effects of gender and age on the levels and circadian rhythmicity of plasma cortisol. J Clin Endocrinol Metab 1996;81: 2468–73.
39. Straub RH, Miller LE, Scholmerich J, et al. Cytokines and hormones as possible links between endocrinosenescence and immunosenescence. J Neuroimmunol 2000;109:10–5.
40. Heuser IJ, Gotthardt U, Schweiger U, et al. Age-associated changes of pituitary-adrenocortical hormone regulation in humans: importance of gender. Neurobiol Aging 1994;15:227–31.
41. Kudielka BM, Schmidt-Reinwald AK, Hellhammer DH, et al. Psychological and endocrine responses to psychosocial stress and dexamethasone/corticotropin-releasing hormone in healthy postmenopausal women and young controls: the impact of age and a two-week estradiol treatment. Neuroendocrinology 1999;70:422–30.
42. Otte C, Hart S, Neylan TC, et al. A meta-analysis of cortisol response to challenge in human aging: importance of gender. Psychoneuroendocrinology 2005;30:80–91.
43. Gotthardt U, Schweiger U, Fahrenberg J, et al. Cortisol, ACTH, and cardiovascular response to a cognitive challenge paradigm in aging and depression. Am J Physiol 1995;268:R865–73.
44. Kudielka BM, Buske-Kirschbaum A, Hellhammer DH, et al. HPA axis responses to laboratory psychosocial stress in healthy elderly adults, younger adults, and children: impact of age and gender. Psychoneuroendocrinology 2004;29:83–98.
45. Rohleder N, Kudielka BM, Hellhammer DH, et al. Age and sex steroid-related changes in glucocorticoid sensitivity of pro-inflammatory cytokine production after psychosocial stress. J Neuroimmunol 2002;126:69–77.
46. Nicolson N, Storms C, Ponds R, et al. Salivary cortisol levels and stress reactivity in human aging. J Gerontol A Biol Sci Med Sci 1997;52:M68–75.
47. Traustadottir T, Bosch PR, Matt KS. The HPA axis response to stress in women: effects of aging and fitness. Psychoneuroendocrinology 2005;30:392–402.
48. Traustadottir T, Bosch PR, Matt KS. Gender differences in cardiovascular and hypothalamic- pituitary-adrenal axis responses to psychological stress in

healthy older adult men and women. Stress: The international journal on the biology of stress 2003;6:133–40.

49. Kudielka BM, Hellhammer DH, Wust S. Why do we respond so differently? Reviewing determinants of human salivary cortisol responses to challenge. Psychoneuroendocrinology 2009;34:2–18.

50. Stroud LR, Salovey P, Epel ES. Sex differences in stress responses: social rejection versus achievement stress. Biol Psychiatry 2002;52:318–27.

51. Heffner KL, Kiecolt-Glaser JK, Loving TJ, et al. Spousal support satisfaction as a modifier of physiological responses to marital conflict in younger and older couples. J Behav Med 2004;27:233–54.

52. Wilkinson CW, Petrie EC, Murray SR, et al. Human glucocorticoid feedback inhibition is reduced in older individuals: evening study. J Clin Endocrinol Metab 2001;86:545–50.

53. Bornstein SR, Engeland WC, Ehrhart-Bornstein M, et al. Dissociation of ACTH and glucocorticoids. Trends Endocrinol Metab 2008;19:175–80.

54. DeRijk RH, Petrides J, Deuster P, et al. Changes in corticosteroid sensitivity of peripheral blood lymphocytes after strenuous exercise in humans. J Clin Endocrinol Metab 1996;81:228–35.

55. Daun JM, Ball RW, Cannon JG. Glucocorticoid sensitivity of interleukin-1 agonist and antagonist secretion: the effects of age and gender. Am J Physiol Regul Integr Comp Physiol 2000;278:R855–62.

56. Miller GE, Chen E, Fok AK, et al. Low early-life social class leaves a biological residue manifested by decreased glucocorticoid and increased proinflammatory signaling. Proc Natl Acad Sci U S A 2009;106:14716–21.

57. Miller GE, Cohen S, Ritchey AK. Chronic psychological stress and the regulation of pro-inflammatory cytokines: a glucocorticoid-resistance model. Health Psychol 2002;21:531–41.

58. Rohleder N, Wolf JM, Kirschbaum C. Glucocorticoid sensitivity in humans-interindividual differences and acute stress effects. Stress 2003;6:207–22.

59. Chrousos GP, Detera-Wadleigh SD, Karl M. Syndromes of glucocorticoid resistance. Ann Intern Med 1993;119:1113–24.

60. Rhen T, Cidlowski JA. Antiinflammatory action of glucocorticoids–new mechanisms for old drugs. N Engl J Med 2005;353:1711–23.

61. Heijnen CJ. Receptor regulation in neuroendocrine-immune communication: current knowledge and future perspectives. Brain Behav Immun 2007;21:1–8.

62. Barnes PJ. Mechanisms and resistance in glucocorticoid control of inflammation. J Steroid Biochem Mol Biol 2010;120(2–3):76–85.

63. Rosewicz S, McDonald AR, Maddux BA, et al. Mechanism of glucocorticoid receptor down-regulation by glucocorticoids. J Biol Chem 1988;263:2581–4.

64. Webster JC, Oakley RH, Jewell CM, et al. Proinflammatory cytokines regulate human glucocorticoid receptor gene expression and lead to the accumulation of the dominant negative beta isoform: a mechanism for the generation of glucocorticoid resistance. Proc Natl Acad Sci U S A 2001;98:6865–70.

65. Agarwal SK, Marshall GD Jr. Dexamethasone promotes type 2 cytokine production primarily through inhibition of type 1 cytokines. J Interferon Cytokine Res 2001;21:147–55.

66. Elenkov IJ, Chrousos GP. Stress hormones, proinflammatory and antiinflammatory cytokines, and autoimmunity. Ann N Y Acad Sci 2002;966:290–303.

67. Buske-Kirschbaum A, Fischbach S, Rauh W, et al. Increased responsiveness of the hypothalamus-pituitary-adrenal (HPA) axis to stress in newborns with atopic disposition. Psychoneuroendocrinology 2004;29:705–11.

68. Wright RJ, Finn P, Contreras JP, et al. Chronic caregiver stress and IgE expression, allergen-induced proliferation, and cytokine profiles in a birth cohort predisposed to atopy. J Allergy Clin Immunol 2004;113:1051–7.
69. Kiecolt-Glaser JK, Heffner KL, Glaser R, et al. How stress and anxiety can alter immediate and late phase skin test responses in allergic rhinitis. Psychoneuroendocrinology 2009;34:670–80.
70. Buske-Kirschbaum A, Geiben A, Hollig H, et al. Altered responsiveness of the hypothalamus-pituitary-adrenal axis and the sympathetic adrenomedullary system to stress in patients with atopic dermatitis. J Clin Endocrinol Metab 2002;87:4245–51.
71. Orentreich N, Brind JL, Rizer RL, et al. Age changes and sex differences in serum dehydroepiandrosterone sulfate concentrations throughout adulthood. J Clin Endocrinol Metab 1984;59:551–5.
72. Orentreich N, Brind JL, Vogelman JH, et al. Long-term longitudinal measurements of plasma dehydroepiandrosterone sulfate in normal men. J Clin Endocrinol Metab 1992;75:1002–4.
73. Vermeulen A. Dehydroepiandrosterone sulfate and aging. Ann N Y Acad Sci 1995;774:121–7.
74. Hornsby PJ. Biosynthesis of DHEAS by the human adrenal cortex and its age-related decline. Ann N Y Acad Sci 1995;774:29–46.
75. Parker CR Jr, Mixon RL, Brissie RM, et al. Aging alters zonation in the adrenal cortex of men. J Clin Endocrinol Metab 1997;82:3898–901.
76. Arlt W, Hewison M. Hormones and immune function: implications of aging. Aging Cell 2004;3:209–16.
77. Kahonen MH, Tilvis RS, Jolkkonen J, et al. Predictors and clinical significance of declining plasma dehydroepiandrosterone sulfate in old age. Aging 2000;12: 308–14.
78. Tannenbaum C, Barrett-Connor E, Laughlin GA, et al. A longitudinal study of dehydroepiandrosterone sulphate (DHEAS) change in older men and women: the rancho bernardo study. Eur J Endocrinol 2004;151:717–25 European federation of endocrine societies.
79. Mazat L, Lafont S, Berr C, et al. Prospective measurements of dehydroepiandrosterone sulfate in a cohort of elderly subjects: relationship to gender, subjective health, smoking habits, and 10-year mortality. Proc Natl Acad Sci U S A 2001;98:8145–50.
80. Izawa S, Sugaya N, Shirotsuki K, et al. Salivary dehydroepiandrosterone secretion in response to acute psychosocial stress and its correlations with biological and psychological changes. Biol Psychol 2008;79:294–8.
81. Morgan CA 3rd, Southwick S, Hazlett G, et al. Relationships among plasma dehydroepiandrosterone sulfate and cortisol levels, symptoms of dissociation, and objective performance in humans exposed to acute stress. Arch Gen Psychiatry 2004;61:819–25.
82. Maninger N, Capitanio JP, Mason WA, et al. Acute and chronic stress increase DHEAS concentrations in rhesus monkeys. Psychoneuroendocrinology 2010; 35(7):1055–62.
83. Parker CR Jr, Slayden SM, Azziz R, et al. Effects of aging on adrenal function in the human: responsiveness and sensitivity of adrenal androgens and cortisol to adrenocorticotropin in premenopausal and postmenopausal women. J Clin Endocrinol Metab 2000;85:48–54.
84. Kalimi M, Shafagoj Y, Loria R, et al. Anti-glucocorticoid effects of dehydroepiandrosterone (DHEA). Mol Cell Biochem 1994;131:99–104.

85. Hechter O, Grossman A, Chatterton RT Jr. Relationship of dehydroepiandrosterone and cortisol in disease. Med Hypotheses 1997;49:85–91.
86. Daynes RA, Araneo BA, Ershler WB, et al. Altered regulation of IL-6 production with normal aging. Possible linkage to the age-associated decline in dehydroepiandrosterone and its sulfated derivative. J Immunol 1993;150:5219–30 (Baltimore Md: 1950).
87. Padgett DA, Loria RM. Endocrine regulation of murine macrophage function: effects of dehydroepiandrosterone, androstenediol, and androstenetriol. J Neuroimmunol 1998;84:61–8.
88. Catania RA, Angele MK, Ayala A, et al. Dehydroepiandrosterone restores immune function following trauma-haemorrhage by a direct effect on T lymphocytes. Cytokine 1999;11:443–50.
89. Suzuki T, Suzuki N, Daynes RA, et al. Dehydroepiandrosterone enhances IL2 production and cytotoxic effector function of human T cells. Clin Immunol Immunopathol 1991;61:202–11.
90. Gordon CM, LeBoff MS, Glowacki J. Adrenal and gonadal steroids inhibit IL-6 secretion by human marrow cells. Cytokine 2001;16:178–86.
91. Loria RM. Beta-androstenes and resistance to viral and bacterial infections. Neuroimmunomodulation 2009;16:88–95.
92. Kovacs EJ, Duffner LA, Plackett TP. Immunosuppression after injury in aged mice is associated with a TH1-TH2 shift, which can be restored by estrogen treatment. Mech Ageing Dev 2004;125:121–3.
93. Kovacs EJ, Plackett TP, Witte PL. Estrogen replacement, aging, and cell-mediated immunity after injury. J Leukoc Biol 2004;76:36–41.
94. Gilliver S. Sex steroids as inflammatory regulators. J Steroid Biochem Mol Biol 2010;120(2–3):105–15.
95. Delpedro AD, Barjavel MJ, Mamdouh Z, et al. Activation of human monocytes by LPS and DHEA. J Interferon Cytokine Res 1998;18:125–35.
96. Khorram O, Vu L, Yen SS. Activation of immune function by dehydroepiandrosterone (DHEA) in age-advanced men. J Gerontol A Biol Sci Med Sci 1997;52:M1–7.
97. Casson PR, Andersen RN, Herrod HG, et al. Oral dehydroepiandrosterone in physiologic doses modulates immune function in postmenopausal women. Am J Obstet Gynecol 1993;169:1536–9.
98. Dillon JS. Dehydroepiandrosterone, dehydroepiandrosterone sulfate and related steroids: their role in inflammatory, allergic and immunological disorders. Curr Drug Targets Inflamm Allergy 2005;4:377–85.
99. Bauer ME, Jeckel CM, Luz C. The role of stress factors during aging of the immune system. Ann N Y Acad Sci 2009;1153:139–52.
100. Esler M, Kaye D, Thompson J, et al. Effects of aging on epinephrine secretion and regional release of epinephrine from the human heart. J Clin Endocrinol Metab 1995;80:435–42.
101. Iwase S, Mano T, Watanabe T, et al. Age-related changes of sympathetic outflow to muscles in humans. J Gerontol 1991;46:M1–5.
102. Christensen NJ, Jensen EW. Effect of psychosocial stress and age on plasma norepinephrine levels: a review. Psychosom Med 1994;56:77–83.
103. Seals DR, Esler MD. Human ageing and the sympathoadrenal system. J Physiol 2000;528:407–17.
104. Ng AV, Callister R, Johnson DG, et al. Age and gender influence muscle sympathetic nerve activity at rest in healthy humans. Hypertension 1993;21:498–503.
105. Kudielka BM, Schmidt-Reinwald AK, Hellhammer DH, et al. Psychosocial stress and HPA functioning: no evidence for a reduced resilience in healthy elderly men. Stress 2000;3:229–40.

106. Esler M, Lambert G, Kaye D, et al. Influence of ageing on the sympathetic nervous system and adrenal medulla at rest and during stress. Biogerontology 2002;3:45–9.
107. Franco-Morselli R, Elghozi JL, Joly E, et al. Increased plasma adrenaline concentrations in benign essential hypertension. Br Med J 1977;2:1251–4.
108. Weidmann P, Beretta-Piccoli C, Ziegler WH, et al. Age versus urinary sodium for judging renin, aldosterone, and catecholamine levels: studies in normal subjects and patients with essential hypertension. Kidney Int 1978;14:619–28.
109. Palmer GJ, Ziegler MG, Lake CR. Response of norepinephrine and blood pressure to stress increases with age. J Gerontol 1978;33:482–7.
110. Aslan S, Nelson L, Carruthers M, et al. Stress and age effects on catecholamines in normal subjects. J Psychosom Res 1981;25:33–41.
111. Mazzeo RS, Rajkumar C, Jennings G, et al. Norepinephrine spillover at rest and during submaximal exercise in young and old subjects. J Appl Physiol 1997;82: 1869–74.
112. Friedman EM, Irwin MR. Modulation of immune cell function by the autonomic nervous system. Pharmacol Ther 1997;74:27–38.
113. Nance DM, Sanders VM. Autonomic innervation and regulation of the immune system (1987–2007). Brain Behav Immun 2007;21:736–45.
114. Callahan TA, Moynihan JA. Contrasting pattern of cytokines in antigen- versus mitogen-stimulated splenocyte cultures from chemically denervated mice. Brain Behav Immun 2002;16:764–73.
115. Salicru AN, Sams CF, Marshall GD. Cooperative effects of corticosteroids and catecholamines upon immune deviation of the type-1/type-2 cytokine balance in favor of type-2 expression in human peripheral blood mononuclear cells. Brain Behav Immun 2007;21:913–20.
116. Straub RH, Cutolo M, Zietz B, et al. The process of aging changes the interplay of the immune, endocrine and nervous systems. Mech Ageing Dev 2001;122: 1591–611.
117. Kiecolt-Glaser JK, Glaser R, Gravenstein S, et al. Chronic stress alters the immune response to influenza virus vaccine in older adults. Proc Natl Acad Sci U S A 1996;93:3043–7.
118. Besedovsky H, Sorkin E, Felix D, et al. Hypothalamic changes during the immune response. Eur J Immunol 1977;7:323–5.
119. Pawelec G, Larbi A, Pawelec G, et al. Immunity and ageing in man: annual review 2006/2007. Exp Gerontol 2008;43:34–8.
120. McEwen BS. Sex, stress and the hippocampus: allostasis, allostatic load and the aging process. Neurobiol Aging 2002;23:921–39.
121. Seeman TE, McEwen BS, Rowe JW, et al. Allostatic load as a marker of cumulative biological risk: MacArthur studies of successful aging. Proc Natl Acad Sci U S A 2001;98:4770–5.

Biobehavioral Influences on Cancer Progression

Erin S. Costanzo, PhD[a],*, Anil K. Sood, MD[b],
Susan K. Lutgendorf, PhD[c]

KEYWORDS

• Cancer • Stress • Depression • Immunity • Inflammation
• Angiogenesis

Epidemiologically documented risk factors for carcinogenesis, including genetic, endocrine, environmental, and socioeconomic factors, only account for part of the risk for cancer initiation.[1] Similarly, patients who have cancer who have a similar prognosis based on known clinical risk factors vary significantly with respect to disease outcomes. Emerging research has focused on the contributions of behavioral factors and neuroendocrine stress response pathways in explaining this individual variation. This area of research stems from epidemiologic and other observational studies showing links between factors such as life stress, depression, social support, and cancer. Evidence for the contribution of behavioral factors to cancer initiation is modest and findings are inconsistent,[2–5] with the most promising work focusing on interactions between behavioral factors and other host factors that may confer vulnerability, such as aging and tobacco use.[6] However, a much stronger literature supports links between behavioral factors and cancer progression once a tumor has been established.[7–18] This review focuses on contributions of behavioral factors to disease progression and potential mechanisms underlying these relationships. We describe behavioral factors that are important in modulation of the stress response and

This work was supported by grants KL2 RR0205012 from the Clinical and Translational Science Award (CTSA) program of the National Center for Research Resources and R21 CA133343 from the National Cancer Institute to ESC, R01 CA140933 and R01 CA104825 from the National Cancer Institute to SKL, and R01 CA110793, RO1 CA109298, and P50 CA083693 (MD Anderson Cancer Center SPORE in Ovarian Cancer) from the National Cancer Institute and a Program Project Development Grant from the Ovarian Cancer Research Fund, Inc to AKS.

[a] Department of Psychiatry, Carbone Comprehensive Cancer Center, University of Wisconsin-Madison, 6001 Research Park Boulevard, Madison, WI 53719, USA
[b] Departments of Gynecologic Oncology, Cancer Biology, and Center for RNA Interference and Non-Coding RNA, MD Anderson Cancer Center, University of Texas, Unit 1362, PO Box 301439, Houston, TX 77230, USA
[c] Departments of Psychology, Urology, Obstetrics & Gynecology, Holden Comprehensive Cancer Center, University of Iowa, E11 Seashore Hall, Iowa City, IA 52242, USA
* Corresponding author.
E-mail address: ecostanzo@wisc.edu

Immunol Allergy Clin N Am 31 (2011) 109–132
doi:10.1016/j.iac.2010.09.001
0889-8561/11/$ – see front matter © 2011 Elsevier Inc. All rights reserved.

the pivotal role of neuroendocrine regulation in the downstream alteration of immune, inflammatory, and tumor physiology. Consequences for cancer growth and progression are delineated, and implications of these findings for behavioral and pharmacologic interventions are discussed.

BIOBEHAVIORAL MODEL OF CANCER CONTROL
Behavioral Factors

Stress is commonly defined as the experience of a negative life event or the occurrence of such an event along with a subjective evaluation of inadequacy to effectively cope with it.[19] Diagnosis with a life-threatening illness such as cancer is almost universally experienced as stressful.[20–22] In addition, cancer diagnosis and treatment are accompanied by several acute and chronic stressors that can affect quality of life. Severe life stress is often associated with the development of depression or anxiety.[23–26] Depression is common among individuals with cancer, with about one-third of patients with cancer reporting depressive symptoms at the time of diagnosis, and up to one-fourth suffering from symptoms sufficient to meet criteria for a clinical diagnosis of major depression.[27,28]

Most behavioral research in cancer has focused on distress and negative emotions, but there has been growing attention to markers of resilience.[29] Social support, frequently defined as the degree of perceived satisfaction with social relationships, is an important psychological resource. It is believed to have direct benefits for psychological and health outcomes and to buffer the effects of stress on mental and physical health.[30–33] High levels of social support have been consistently associated with diminished risk for morbidity and mortality, with statistical effect sizes comparable with those of standard health risk factors such as smoking, blood pressure, cholesterol, obesity, and exercise.[34] Additional resilience factors, including optimism and the ability to find meaning or perceive some benefit in one's experience with cancer, are discussed in this article.

Although health practices such as diet, exercise, and tobacco use are also classified as behavior, these influences have already been characterized in other literatures. The current review focuses on the roles of psychological and social factors in cancer progression. A model of biobehavioral processes relevant to cancer control is illustrated in **Fig. 1**.

Neuroendocrine Stress Response Pathways

External events evaluated as threatening or stressful activate cortical and limbic structures of the central nervous system and ultimately activate the hypothalamic pituitary adrenocortical (HPA) axis and sympathetic nervous system.[35] Specifically, corticotrophin-releasing hormone and vasopressin are secreted from the paraventricular nucleus of the hypothalamus in response to psychological stress or other affective experiences. These neurohormones stimulate the anterior pituitary to produce adrenocorticotrophic hormone, which in turn stimulates the release of the glucocorticoid hormone cortisol from the adrenal glands. The sympathetic nervous system (SNS) is known for its role in the fight-or-flight stress response. Sympathetic fibers innervate the adrenal medulla, releasing acetylcholine, which activates the secretion of epinephrine (E) and norepinephrine (NE). SNS fibers also directly innervate many tissues, including primary and secondary lymphoid tissue where they are involved in the regulation of the immune response. Glucocorticoids, catecholamines, and other neuroendocrine factors have been shown to have modulatory effects on immune processes relevant to tumor surveillance and containment, as well as on other pathophysiologic processes important in cancer progression, including angiogenesis, invasion, and modulation of inflammation.[6,36–38] These pathways and their translational implications are discussed later.

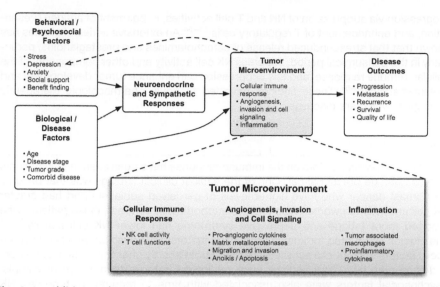

Fig. 1. In addition to known biomedical risk factors, this biobehavioral model of cancer control illustrates the contributions of behavioral risk and resilience factors to cancer outcomes. Stress-related behavioral factors can activate (or inhibit) the hypothalamic pituitary adrenocortical (HPA) axis and sympathetic nervous systems (SNS). The products of these pathways, including glucocorticoids, catecholamines, and other neuroendocrine factors, have downstream effects on physiologic mechanisms in the tumor micorenvironment that are important for the control of malignancy. These effects include the modulation of cellular immune processes relevant to tumor surveillance and containment, inflammation, and other pathophysiologic processes critical to cancer growth and progression, including angiogenesis, invasion, and tumor-promoting cell signaling pathways. Alteration of these physiologic processes can encourage or inhibit tumor progression and metastasis. The potential effects of tumor- and treatment-derived inflammatory processes on depression (*dashed arrow*) and quality of life are also illustrated.

BIOBEHAVIORAL PATHWAYS: IMMUNOSUPPRESSION

Modulating effects of behavioral factors on the cellular immune response via activation of the HPA and SNS have been well characterized,[39–41] with mechanisms including direct sympathetic innervation of immune tissue, presence of glucocorticoid and β-adrenergic receptors on mononuclear leukocytes, and neuroendocrine modification of lymphocyte trafficking.[37,40,42,43] Psychological stress and affective responses, including depression and anxiety, have been associated with downregulation of cellular immune responses, including the number and type of lymphocytes in circulation, proliferative and cytolytic responses in vitro, and antibody levels after immunization.[44,45] These findings are believed to have relevance to cancer control because of the potential role of cellular immunity, particularly natural killer (NK) cell activity, in the defense against malignant cells.[46,47] The underlying assumption of the immunosuppression model is that stress or negative emotions can modulate tumor initiation and development by suppressing elements of the immune response important in responding to malignant cells.[22,36,48–50]

Preclinical Studies

Preclinical experimental studies have documented that chronic stress, as well as significant acute stress associated with surgery, promote tumor incidence and progression via suppression of NK and T cell activities, impairment of antigen presentation, and enhancement of T regulatory cells.[51–54] An extensive series of studies has shown that that stress-induced release of catecholamines and prostaglandins, particularly in the perisurgical period, suppress NK cell activity and other components of the cellular immune response, and this suppression can enhance tumor development and metastasis.[52,53,55–57] These findings have led to novel pharmacologic therapeutic strategies, which are discussed later.

Clinical Studies

Effects of behavioral factors on the immune response have been examined in patients with early-stage breast cancer. One of the earliest clinical findings was that patients with breast cancer who have higher levels of perceived social support had greater NK cell activity than women who felt less supported. In contrast, those patients who reported more fatigue and depressive symptoms had lower NK cell activity.[58–61] The studies accounted for known prognostic factors; relationships between psychosocial factors and NK cell activity were found both shortly after breast cancer surgery and 3 months later, and findings were replicated in more than 1 patient sample. Psychosocial factors were also associated with time to recurrence; however, NK cell activity was not found to mediate the links between psychosocial factors and recurrence.[62]

These findings have been extended in a more recent series of studies involving a large sample of patients with breast cancer followed for 18 months after surgery. After accounting for the relevant clinical factors, women who reported greater distress after surgery showed a diminished cellular immune response across a variety of measures including less robust NK cell activity, poorer response of NK cells to recombinant IFNγ, a decreased lymphoproliferative response, and altered expression of inhibitory NK cell receptors.[20,63] Moreover, patients who displayed more rapid reductions in distress after surgery also showed the fastest recovery of NK cell activity over time.[64] Other recent studies provide additional evidence for links between psychosocial factors and alteration of markers of cellular immunity, including NK cell count and activity, lymphoproliferative responses, and B and T cell subsets in patients with breast cancer[65–69] as well as among patients with other types of cancers, including gynecologic, prostate, gastrointestinal, digestive tract, and liver malignancies.[70–74] Whereas most research has focused on markers of stress and maladjustment and downregulation of cellular immunity, recent work has also attended to processes of resilience that may optimize immune function. For example, among women with early-stage breast cancer, a greater ability to find benefit in one's experience with cancer was associated with a better lymphoproliferative response.[68] Similarly, men with localized prostate cancer who were more optimistic and were able to more adaptively express their anger showed better NK cell cytotoxicity.[72]

Despite the accumulating evidence that the psychological state of patients who have cancer can alter cellular immunity, not all findings have been consistent,[75] and effects on cellular immune markers have varied.[64,67,76] Moreover, the implications of these relationships for clinical end points including disease recurrence and survival have been difficult to investigate because of the large sample size and long follow-up required. A recent report showed that patients with hepatobiliary carcinoma who exceeded a cutoff score that indicates clinically significant depressive symptomatology showed lower NK cell numbers and shorter survival compared with their nondepressed counterparts. Moreover, the investigators found that NK cell count mediated the relationship between depression and survival.[9]

There has been increasing attention to immune markers in the tumor microenvironment, where the potential for clinical significance may be greater. For example, studies of patients with ovarian cancer examined cellular immune functioning in both peripheral blood and in tumor infiltrating lymphocytes (TIL). Distress was associated with poorer NK cell activity and lower TH_1/TH_2 cell ratios both in peripheral blood and in TIL. In contrast, social support was associated with greater NK cell activity in TIL and a greater percentage of NKT cells in tumor ascites.[74,76,77]

The immunosupression model has not been able to consistently account for links between behavioral factors and cancer outcomes, suggesting some limitations of this model in the biobehavioral context. Tumors have escape mechanisms by which they evade recognition and destruction by the immune response, including downregulation of class I major histocompatability complex (MHC-I) and tumor-associated antigens, interference with costimulatory signals, and disruption of apoptotic signaling. Interactions of stress pathways with tumor escape mechanisms have been minimally investigated and may prove to be an area of great potential. In addition, there are other mechanisms by which stress and psychological responses can influence the tumor microenvironment and the growth and progression of malignancies.

BIOBEHAVIORAL PATHWAYS: ANGIOGENESIS, INVASION, AND CELL SIGNALING
Malignant Transformation, Angiogenesis, and Metastasis

Tumors are complex tissues that are shaped by ongoing interactions between cancer cells and the surrounding microenvironment.[78–80] Many of the steps involved in malignant cell transformation and metastasis involve signaling interactions with surrounding cells that may be induced by tumor cells to secrete molecules supporting abnormal development, proliferation, and angiogenesis.[81–83] After the initial transformation and proliferation, vascularization of the tumor mass is critical for its growth and metastatic spread.[84,85] This process, referred to as angiogenesis, is normally tightly controlled by positive and negative factors secreted by both tumor and host cells.[85,86] Proangiogenic molecules include vascular endothelial growth factor (VEGF), interleukin-6 (IL-6), and interleukin-8 (IL-8). During tumor development, an angiogenic switch is triggered whereby the balance of angiogenic inducers and inhibiters changes, and angiogenesis proceeds.[81] After an adequate blood supply has been established, tumor cells invade the host tissues and the cancer grows locally.[87] The process of metastasis involves detachment and embolization of tumor cells, which travel through the circulation, arrest in the capillary beds of specific organs, and ultimately establish a new microenvironment at that site.[87]

Stress-based Modulation of Angiogenesis

Increasing evidence has shown that behavioral and neuroendocrine factors can modulate the tumor growth pathways described earlier.[88–96] In vitro studies have shown that tumor production of VEGF is stimulated by stress-related mediators such as NE, E, and cortisol in ovarian cancer, melanoma, and nasopharyngeal cancer cell lines. This occurs via β-adrenergic signaling and is blocked by the β-blocker propanolol.[93,94,97] Preclinical experiments with an orthotopic model of ovarian cancer have shown that chronic restraint stress increases tumor weight and number of tumor nodules. These effects were mediated by increases in VEGF and angiogenesis induced by β-adrenergic pathways, could be replicated by the β-adrenergic agonist isoproterenol, and were blocked by propranolol.[91] Similarly, surgical stress increased ovarian tumor growth in an orthotopic animal model via β-adrenergically linked angiogenic pathways, with the stress effects reversed by β-adrenergic blockage.[98] Parallel findings have been observed in the clinical setting, where social isolation among women with ovarian cancer has been linked to higher levels of VEGF both in serum taken at the time of surgery and in tumor tissue.[96,99]

Behavioral factors and stress response pathways can also modulate other cytokines involved in angiogenesis. Interleukin-6 (IL-6) is produced by tumor cells and tumor-associated macrophages (TAM) and plays multiple roles in tumor progression, including a key role in angiogenesis.[100,101] IL-6 also stimulates proliferation of tumor cells,[102,103] enhances tumor cell migration and attachment,[103] promotes invasion of endothelial cells,[104] and is associated with tumor progression and poorer clinical outcomes.[105–107] Of relevance to biobehavioral pathways, IL-6 is regulated by neural and endocrine stress responses via feedback loops with the HPA axis.[108–110] Moreover, IL-6 levels are increased with sympathetic activation, acute and chronic stress, and depression.[95,108,109,111–116] Increases of IL-6 in both plasma and ascites within the tumor compartment have been observed in patient with ovarian cancer with greater social isolation, suggesting the potential clinical relevance of social interactions.[117] Interleukin-8 (IL-8) is another proangiogenic molecule induced by various stressors in humans.[118,119] In vitro, NE has been shown to stimulate IL-6 gene transcription through an Src-dependent mechanism and has increased IL-8 secretion in cancer cell lines, showing effects of stress mechanisms on critical tumor signaling pathways.[90,95,116]

In addition to activation of proangiogenic cytokines such as VEGF and IL-6, stress response pathways have been shown to directly activate angiogenesis-promoting molecules such as signal transducer and activator of transcription factor-3 (STAT-3). Stimulation by NE and E can activate STAT-3 independently of IL-6, leading to its downstream effects on cell proliferation, survival, and angiogenesis, as well as inhibition of apoptosis.[120]

Invasion and Migration

Stress hormones have also been shown to modulate migration and invasion of malignant cells by stimulating production of matrix metalloproteineases (MMP) by both tumor and stromal cells, and by serving as chemoattractants, inducing cell migration. For example, stimulation by NE and E significantly increased ovarian cancer cell production of MMP-2 and MMP-9 through the β-adrenergic signaling pathway.[89] Similar enhancement of MMP production by catecholamines has also been reported in colon and head and neck cancers.[94,121–123] Both NE and cortisol have been shown to enhance MMP-9 production by human monocyte-derived macrophages in vitro.[124] Incubation with levels of NE commensurate with those that would be observed in the organ microenvironment during stress responses significantly increased the invasive potential of ovarian cancer cells, an effect that was reversed by the β-antagonist propranolol.[89]

Recent findings have shown that β-adrenergic signaling promotes survival of ovarian cancer cells by inhibiting anoikis, the normal process of apoptosis that occurs when cells are separated from the extracellular matrix.[92] Resistance to anoikis is a key feature of malignant transformation and enhances the ability of tumor cells to migrate and metastasize to secondary sites. This process occurs through β-adrenergic activation of focal adhesion kinase (FAK) and was seen both in vitro and in an orthotopic mouse model of ovarian cancer. In patients with ovarian cancer, higher levels of pFAK^{Y397} were observed in patients with higher levels of depression or greater NE levels in their tumors. Furthermore, pFAK^{Y397} was linked to poorer overall survival.[92] These data indicate that stress-related FAK modulation may contribute to tumor progression.

Behavioral Factors and Gene Regulation

Psychosocial profiles have also been linked to regulation of gene expression in ovarian cancer. Tumors from patients with ovarian cancer with high levels of depression and low social support (high risk) were compared with those with low levels of depression and high social support (low risk) after being matched for age, grade, stage, and tumor histology. Genome-wide transcriptional analysis and promoter-based bioinformatics analyses were used for tumor profiling. Compared with low-risk patients, tumors from high-risk patients showed more than 200 upregulated gene transcripts and increased activity of signaling pathways involved in tumor growth and progression (eg, CREB/ATF, NFKB/Rel, STAT, and ETS-family transcription factors). High-risk patients also showed increased intratumoral NE levels.[125] These findings suggest that biobehavioral processes may regulate gene expression profiles within solid tumors. β-Adrenergic transcription control pathways seem to be key candidates in mediation of these effects.

In sum, this emerging body of research provides compelling evidence that behavioral factors and stress response pathways are associated with key elements involved in tumor growth and development.

BIOBEHAVIORAL PATHWAYS: INFLAMMATION
Inflammation and Cancer: The Role of Macrophages

Inflammation is a common characteristic of epithelial tumors and serves as a tumor initiator and promoter.[80] TAM are a major contributor to inflammation and constitute a large proportion of most tumor microenvironments.[126] Drawn by tumor-derived chemotactic factors produced by tumors, peripheral monocytes are recruited to the tumor microenvironment, where they differentiate into macrophages. In the presence of a proinflammatory tumor microenvironment, macrophages are induced to switch from their phagocytic (M1) phenotype to an M2 phenotype that produces immunosuppressive cytokines such as IL-10 and TGFβ, key tumor-promoting molecules such as VEGF and MMPs, and some inflammatory cytokines.[83,127,128] TAM are thus directly involved in the following processes: (1) stimulation of angiogenesis; (2) stimulation of tumor proliferation, invasion, and metastases; (3) promotion of degradation and remodeling of the extracellular matrix; and (4) downregulation of the adaptive immune response.[127,129–131] Extensive TAM infiltration is therefore associated with poorer survival.[132–134]

Biobehavioral and Neuroendocrine Modulation of Inflammation

Links between distress, depression, and inflammatory responses have been well documented, with relationships believed to be mediated by HPA dysregulation.[135,136] Relationships between psychosocial factors and proinflammatory and proangiogenic cytokines have been observed in patients with cancer, as reviewed earlier.[96,99,117] Inflammation in the tumor microenvironment is mediated by both tumor cells and immune cells such as macrophages. Behavioral factors such as stress and depression may contribute to enhanced tumor cell secretion of proinflammatory cytokines; for example, NE stimulates IL-6 expression by ovarian cancer cells.[95] Macrophages contain both α- and β-adrenergic receptors, and catecholamines have been shown to promote macrophage production of proinflammatory cytokines such as IL-1β and TNFα, as well as MMP-9.[136–139] Clinically, high levels of chronic stress, depression, and social isolation have been associated with TAM production of MMP-9 in patients with ovarian cancer,[124] suggesting that behavioral factors can alter the tumor microenvironment in a way that favors cancer progression. Behavioral factors have also been shown to affect transcriptional regulation of pathways relevant to inflammation and inflammatory control. For example, older adults with high levels of social isolation had profiles that indicated poorer control of inflammation, including impaired transcription of glucocorticoid response genes and increased activity of proinflammatory transcription control pathways in peripheral leukocytes.[140] Taken together, these findings indicate that macrophages and malignant cells are sensitive to neuroendocrine stress hormones in ways that may affect production of molecules that enhance tumor growth and decrease immune effectiveness.

BIDIRECTIONAL PATHWAYS: EFFECTS OF INFLAMMATION ON DEPRESSION AND QUALITY OF LIFE

The discussion thus far has focused on the role of behavioral factors in modulating inflammatory processes relevant to cancer control. However, it is also known that tumor- or treatment-induced peripheral proinflammatory cytokines can activate central nervous system pathways, evoking a syndrome of behavioral and affective responses that has come to be called sickness behaviors because they mimic flulike vegetative symptoms. There are several pathways mediating the effects of peripheral proinflammatory cytokines on the central nervous system, including passage through regions of permeability of the blood-brain barrier and stimulation of afferent fibers in the vagus nerve.[141–144] In the central nervous system, these pathways induce behavioral and affective symptoms such as depressed mood, fatigue, anorexia, impaired concentration, sleep disturbance, enhanced pain sensitivity, and reduced activity.[142,144,145]

Although it has been commonly assumed that the high prevalence of depression among patients with cancer is a reaction to the stress associated with a potentially life-threatening diagnosis and cancer treatment,[146] it has also been hypothesized that inflammatory processes produced secondary to treatment or tumor growth may contribute to the pathogenesis of depression, as well as fatigue and debility, in patients with cancer.[124,147,148] Several studies have documented associations between increased proinflammatory cytokines and depression among patients with cancer.[124,147–150] Similarly, a series of studies has shown that fatigued breast cancer survivors have higher levels of inflammatory markers such as serum interleukin-1 receptor antagonist (IL-1ra), tumor necrosis factor receptor II (TNFRII), and neopterin, lower levels of serum cortisol, flatter diurnal cortisol slopes, and both enhanced inflammatory responses and blunted cortisol responses to an experimental psychological stressor.[151–153] Specific cytokine gene polymorphisms seem to underlie persistent fatigue in patients with breast cancer such that patients showing homozygosity for either variant of the IL-6 174 genotype or the presence of at least 1 cytosine at the IL-1 B-511 locus are more likely to be fatigued.[154] Cortisol dysregulation, particularly increases in evening cortisol levels, has also been linked to fatigue and debility in patients with ovarian cancer.[150] Taken together, these finding suggest that tumor- and treatment-derived proinflammatory cytokines, as well as inflammatory cytokine polymorphisms, contribute to a chronic state of inflammation, ultimately resulting in the emergence of sickness behaviors and dysregulation of the HPA axis.[124]

TRANSLATIONAL IMPLICATIONS: BEHAVIORAL AND PHARMACOLOGIC INTERVENTIONS

Behavioral interventions for patients with cancer, including psychoeducational support groups and psychotherapy, can reduce anxiety, depression, and cancer-related distress and improve quality of life.[155–158] The evidence reviewed thus far also points to the potential for behavioral interventions that can reduce stress and mood disturbance to serve an adjunctive role to conventional treatments in improving outcomes for patients with cancer. An early behavioral intervention trial found that women with metastatic breast cancer randomized to a year-long weekly support group survived an average of 18 months longer than women assigned to a control group.[159,160] However, there has been significant controversy about the meaning of the results (eg, Refs.[161–163]), and attempts to replicate in other samples of patients with breast cancer have not been successful.[164–169] Results from studies of other behavioral interventions have also been mixed. Although several trials have shown no survival effect,[170–172] 3 randomized clinical trials have shown positive results.[160,173–176] One of the most striking findings was that an average of 7 hours of supportive psychotherapy improved survival among patients undergoing surgery for gastrointestinal malignancies, effects that were sustained at 2- and 10-year follow-ups.[174,175]

Such findings have catalyzed interest in the potential mechanisms by which behavioral interventions could affect cancer outcomes. Most studies have focused on the roles of NK cell activity, lymphocyte proliferative response, and other markers cellular immune functioning. There is evidence from a handful of large, well-designed, randomized clinical trials that behavioral interventions that enhance social support and target stress management and other coping skills can improve neuroendocrine and cellular immune functioning.

For example, cognitive-behavioral stress management (CBSM) is a 10-session behavioral program conducted in a supportive group format that assists patients in developing coping skills, using social support, expressing emotions, and learning relaxation strategies. CBSM reduced anxiety and depression and appeared to normalize neuroendocrine functioning in patients with breast cancer; women randomized to the intervention displayed a significant decline in cortisol in a 12-month follow-up period, whereas women in the control group did not show this decline.[158,177–179] CBSM participants also showed better lymphoproliferative responses at a 3-month follow-up and better Th1 responses at a 6-month follow-up, as indicated by greater Th1 cytokine production (IL-2 and IFNγ) and a higher IL-2/IL-4 ratio; however, these differences were not sustained at a 12-month follow-up.[68,179] The effect of CBSM on clinical outcomes has not yet been reported.

Another behavioral intervention that was provided in a supportive group format and targeted coping skills, stress management, health practices, and adherence to treatment showed similar benefits for women with early-stage breast cancer in a randomized clinical trial. In addition to reducing distress and improving social support, the intervention also appeared to be protective with respect to immune functioning. T cell proliferative responses to phytohemagglutinin and concanavalin A remained stable or increased during the 4-month intervention period for participants randomized to the intervention, but declined during the same period for women in the control group, an effect that was maintained at a 12-month follow-up.[180,181] Women who reported clinically significant depressive symptoms were especially likely to benefit; in addition to improvements in mood and quality of life, they also showed reductions in markers of inflammation (operationalized as white blood cell count, neutrophil count, and T helper/T suppressor cell ratio).[182] The intervention also improved clinical outcomes, including initial benefits in performance status, functional status, and overall health status.[181] Perhaps the most notable finding was that, after a median of 11 years of follow-up, women randomized to the psychological intervention showed a reduced risk of breast cancer recurrence and mortality.[173] The investigators plan to investigate whether improvements in cellular immune functioning or reduced inflammation in the intervention participants may be responsible for the survival differences.

A key component of these interventions seems to be the acquisition of specific skills to reduce the effects of stress, both psychologically and physiologically. Mindfulness-based Stress Reduction (MBSR) is an 8-week program that includes several such skills including mindfulness meditation, gentle yoga, and progressive muscle relaxation techniques. MBSR has shown promising effects in patients with cancer, including reduced distress, improved quality of life, declines in cortisol, enhanced NK cell functioning, and a quicker restoration of the balance of Th1 to Th2 cytokines to pretreatment levels.[183–186] Other work has shown benefits from brief training in relaxation techniques and guided imagery, including decreased cortisol; greater numbers of mature and activated T cells, NK cells, and lymphokine-activated killer subsets; improved NK cell activity; and enhanced lymphocyte proliferative responses.[187–191]

Effects of psychosocial interventions on cellular immune functioning have not been found in all studies,[192–194] and the findings have not been uniformly positive in the studies reviewed earlier, with effects shown for some parameters of immune functioning but not others. Nonetheless, there is compelling evidence from at least 2 large, randomized clinical trials for patients with breast cancer that behavioral interventions can optimize cortisol regulation and cellular immune functioning. Follow-up work is needed to replicate and extend these findings, to examine effects of behavioral interventions on tumor growth pathways described earlier, and to determine whether the changes in physiology are of the type and magnitude necessary to alter clinical outcomes.

Targeting specific quality-of-life concerns, such as insomnia, is another promising avenue.[145] For example, a cognitive-behavioral intervention for chronic insomnia among patients with early-stage breast cancer not only improved sleep and fatigue but also increased interferon-γ and IL-1β from before to after treatment, with IL-1β changes maintained at a 1-year follow-up, effects the investigators characterized as immune enhancing. Lymphocyte counts also increased from after treatment to later follow-up time points.[195] Interventions focusing on sleep have the potential to modulate disease-induced alterations in circadian rhythms, which have been closely linked to neuroendocrine and immune regulation relevant to tumor growth.[196,197]

Pharmacologic interventions that can modulate the stress response pathways described in this review also hold promise. There is already evidence that selective serotonin reuptake inhibitors can be effective in addressing cancer-related quality-of-life symptoms.[198,199] The role of antidepressants on tumor growth outcomes has been mixed, with both positive and negative effects reported, depending on the population and the antidepressant.[200,201] Based on evidence that stress-induced alterations in the tumor microenvironment seem to be mediated by β-adrenergic signaling pathways, β-blockers have been proposed as a potential therapeutic strategy to attenuate these effects. β-Blockers have already been shown to reduce the effects of stress on suppression of NK cell activity and tumor development in animal models,[202,203] and there is epidemiologic evidence that β-blocker use reduces risk for the development of prostate cancer in humans.[204] Pilot clinical studies to examine the potential preventative effects of β-blockers are underway. Along similar lines, an innovative cocktail of catecholamine- and prostaglandin-blockers has been successfully used in an animal syngeneic tumor model along with the immunostimulant poly-I-C to prevent perioperative immunosuppression.[205]

FUTURE DIRECTIONS: SENSITIVE POPULATIONS AND WINDOWS OF OPPORTUNITY

The emerging body of literature provides compelling evidence that stress-related behavioral factors can modulate physiologic pathways relevant to cancer control. Because cancers are heterogeneous both in physiology and in treatment, it is important to determine whether the biobehavioral relationships documented in patients with breast and ovarian cancer are seen with other cancer sites and with varying disease burdens. For example, it has been proposed that hormonally mediated malignancies, such prostate and endometrial cancers, may follow similar patterns. Immune-mediated cancers, such as leukemias and lymphomas, also have the potential to be susceptible to the types of behavioral influences reviewed in this article.[180]

Increased attention to clinical significance will be critical in translating findings to meaningful treatments and outcomes. In the past, it has been difficult to assess recurrence and survival because of the large sample sizes and long follow-up period required, but continued efforts in this direction are needed. Studies should also include other clinical end points relevant to morbidity and quality of life, as well as intermediate markers of disease processes. For example, the development of opportunistic infections following immunosuppressive therapy is an outcome that has relevance to quality of life, health care use, and survival. Other treatment complications, such as neutropenia and pancytopenia, can also greatly affect quality of life, may require additional intervention, and can delay therapy. Tumor markers used as an index of disease processes or response to treatment, such as CA125 in ovarian cancer, can easily be assessed even with a brief follow-up period.

We have previously recommended focusing on windows of opportunity in the disease and treatment trajectory that may be most sensitive to the effects of biobehavioral influences.[6] For example, behavioral factors may be most likely to influence immune functioning in a clinically significant way early in the development of the tumor as opposed to once the tumor is well established and sophisticated tumor escape mechanisms have developed. The perioperative period has been proposed to be another critical time period because of the simultaneous occurrence of several risk factors for progression and metastasis, including increased angiogenesis, secretion of growth factors, shedding of tumor cells, and suppression of cellular immunity.[55,203,206] Following surgery, a small number of circulating cancer cells termed minimal residual disease (MRD) can remain and are believed to be the source of disease recurrence in some patients. Indices of cellular immune functioning, including leukocyte cytotoxicity and proliferative responses during this period, predict better clinical outcomes.[203,207,208] Similarly, the recovery from immunosuppressive adjuvant treatment is likely to be another sensitive window. Following adjuvant therapy, MRD is also known to cause relapse, particularly for individuals with hematologic malignancies. The immune system must recover sufficiently to both recognize and destroy remaining malignant cells and to protect against secondary infections.

Hematopoietic Stem Cell Transplantation

Hematopoietic stem cell transplantation (HSCT) provides an illustrative example of some of these ideas. HSCT is a potentially curative, but rigorous, therapy with significant risk of morbidity and mortality. Patients with hematologic malignancies undergoing this treatment frequently experience physical and psychological sequelae that impair their quality of life and undermine recovery. Common adverse physical symptoms include nausea, fatigue, and mucositis as well as the serious complications of persistent infections.[209,210] In addition, 40% to 70% of patients relapse following autologous stem cell transplantation,[211] and graft-versus-host disease is a common and potentially lethal complication of allogeneic transplantation and a cause of significant long-term disability. Many patients therefore report significant emotional distress.[212]

Depressed mood and low levels of hope before HSCT have predicted poorer survival after transplant.[213–216] Biobehavioral pathways important to the control of hematologic malignancies and transplant complications could play a critical mediating role in this setting. As reviewed in this article, it is now widely accepted that many of the host- or recipient-derived cells essential to the recovery of hematopoiesis and immune competence also express receptors for the soluble and cellular factors that are responsive to the extensive cross talk between psychological state and the neuroendocrine and immune systems. These interactions may be of particular significance for patients having HSCT because any modulatory influence on immune processes could have a salient effect on relapse and survival. Immune reconstitution following transplant is directly associated with reduced relapse risk and overall and progression-free survival.[211,217–219] In addition to the potential effects on MRD, recovery of immune competence is also critical for minimizing tissue damage and providing protection against bacterial and viral pathogens.[219]

A related potential application of biobehavioral research in cancer focuses on adoptive immunotherapy, which involves the cultivation of the patient's leukocytes with IL-2 to expand a population of lymphokine-activated killer (LAK) cells known to have antitumor activity. This treatment has been used in melanoma and renal cell carcinoma, as well as after HSCT to boost activity against MRD. Although speculative, the central role of the cellular immune response in the success of both HSCT and adoptive immunotherapy provides an opportunity for biobehavioral factors to influence treatment outcomes.

SUMMARY

Accumulating evidence suggests the importance of considering behavioral risk factors in the care of patients with cancer. Although delineation of mechanisms is still ongoing, there is compelling evidence that behavioral and psychosocial factors that activate the neuroendocrine stress response can alter immune, angiogenic, and inflammatory pathways important in the development, progression, and control of malignancy. Alongside conventional therapies, behavioral interventions incorporating cognitive-behavioral, mindfulness, supportive, and stress management approaches, as well as novel pharmacologic strategies targeting stress response pathways, have the potential to improve the care, well-being, and survival of individuals with cancer.

REFERENCES

1. Daly M, Obrams GI. Epidemiology and risk assessment for ovarian cancer. Semin Oncol 1998;25(3):255–64.
2. Geyer S. Life events prior to manifestation of breast cancer: a limited prospective study covering eight years before diagnosis. J Psychosom Res 1991; 35(2–3):355–63.
3. Duijts SFA, Zeegers MPA, Borne BV. The association between stressful life events and breast cancer risk: a meta-analysis. Int J Cancer 2003;107(6): 1023–9.
4. Lillberg K, Verkasalo PK, Kaprio J, et al. Stressful life events and risk of breast cancer in 10,808 women: a cohort study. Am J Epidemiol 2003;157(5):415–23.
5. Michael YL, Carlson NE, Chlebowski RT, et al. Influence of stressors on breast cancer incidence in the Women's Health Initiative. Health Psychol 2009;28(2):137–46.
6. Lutgendorf SK, Costanzo ES, Siegel S. Psychosocial influences in oncology: an expanded model of biobehavioral mechanisms. In: Ader R, editor. Psychoneuroimmunology. 4th edition. San Diego (CA): Elsevier Academic Press; 2007. p. 869–96.

7. Palesh O, Butler LD, Koopman C, et al. Stress history and breast cancer recurrence. J Psychosom Res 2007;63(3):233–9.
8. Satin JR, Linden W, Phillips MJ. Depression as a predictor of disease progression and mortality in cancer patients: a meta-analysis. Cancer 2009;115(22):5349–61.
9. Steel JL, Geller DA, Gamblin TC, et al. Depression, immunity, and survival in patients with hepatobiliary carcinoma. J Clin Oncol 2007;25(17):2397–405.
10. Petticrew M, Bell R, Hunter D. Influence of psychological coping on survival and recurrence in people with cancer: systematic review. Br Med J 2002;325(7372): 1066–76.
11. Stommel M, Given BA, Given CW. Depression and functional status as predictors of death among cancer patients. Cancer 2002;94(10):2719–27.
12. Epping-Jordan J, Compas B, Howell D. Predictors of cancer progression in young adult men and women: avoidance, intrusive thoughts, and psychological symptoms. Health Psychol 1994;13(6):539–47.
13. Brown JE, Butow PN, Culjak G, et al. Psychosocial predictors of outcome: time to relapse and survival in patients with early stage melanoma. Br J Cancer 2000; 83(11):1448–53.
14. Ell K, Nishimoto R, Mediansky L, et al. Social relations, social support, and survival among patients with cancer. J Psychosom Res 1992;36(6):531–41.
15. Maunsell E, Brisson J, Deschenes L. Social support and survival among women with breast cancer. Cancer 1995;76(4):631–7.
16. Waxler-Morrison N, Hislop TG, Mears B, et al. Effects of social relationships on survival for women with breast cancer: a prospective study. Soc Sci Med 1991; 33(2):177–83.
17. Kroenke CH, Kubzansky LD, Schernhammer ES, et al. Social networks, social support, and survival after breast cancer diagnosis. J Clin Oncol 2006;24(7): 1105–11.
18. Chida Y, Hamer M, Wardle J, et al. Do stress-related psychosocial factors contribute to cancer incidence and survival? Nat Clin Pract Oncol 2008;5(8): 466–75.
19. Lazarus R, Folkman S. Stress, appraisal, and coping. New York: Springer; 1984.
20. Andersen B, Farrar WB, Golden-Kreutz D, et al. Stress and immune responses after surgical treatment for regional breast cancer. J Natl Cancer Inst 1998; 90(1):30–6.
21. Meyerowitz B. Psychosocial correlates of breast cancer and its treatments. Psychol Bull 1980;87(1):108–31.
22. Andersen B, Kiecolt-Glaser J, Glaser R. A biobehavioral model of cancer stress and disease course. Am Psychol 1994;49(5):389–404.
23. Monroe SM, Slavich GM, Torres LD, et al. Severe life events predict specific patterns of change in cognitive biases in major depression. Psychol Med 2007;37(6):863–71.
24. Monroe SM, Slavich GM, Torres LD, et al. Major life events and major chronic difficulties are differentially associated with history of major depressive episodes. J Abnorm Psychol 2007;116(1):116–24.
25. Monroe SM, Harkness KL. Life stress, the "kindling" hypothesis, and the recurrence of depression: considerations from a life stress perspective. Psychol Rev 2005;112(2):417–45.
26. Becker J, Kleinman A. Psychosocial aspects of depression. Hillsdale (NJ): Erlbaum; 1991.
27. Massie MJ. Prevalence of depression in patients with cancer. J Natl Cancer Inst Monogr 2004;32:57–71.

28. Spoletini I, Gianni W, Repetto L, et al. Depression and cancer: an unexplored and unresolved emergent issue in elderly patients. Crit Rev Oncol Hematol 2008;65(2):143–55.

29. Costanzo ES, Ryff CD, Singer B. Psychosocial adjustment among cancer survivors: findings from a national survey of health and well-being. Health Psychol 2009;28:147–56.

30. Cohen S, Wills T. Stress, social support, and the buffering hypothesis. Psychol Bull 1985;98(2):310–57.

31. Cohen S, Underwood LG, Gottlieb BH, editors. Social support measurement and intervention. New York: Oxford University Press; 2000.

32. Cutrona C, Russell D. Type of social support and specific stress: toward a theory of optimal matching. In: Sarason BR, Sarason IG, Pierce GR, editors. Social support: an interactional view. New York: Wiley; 1990. p. 319–66.

33. Cornwell EY, Waite LJ. Social disconnectedness, perceived isolation, and health among older adults. J Health Soc Behav 2009;50(1):31–48.

34. House JS, Landis KR, Umberson D. Social relationships and health. Science 1988;241(4865):540–5.

35. Weiner H. Perturbing the organism: the biology of stressful experience. Chicago: University of Chicago Press; 1992.

36. Antoni M, Lutgendorf S, Cole S, et al. The influence of bio-behavioural factors on tumor biology: pathways and mechanisms. Nat Rev Cancer 2006;6(3):240–8.

37. Madden K. Catcholamines, sympathetic innervation, and immunity. Brain Behav Immun 2003;17:S5–10.

38. Felten DL, Felten SY. Innervation of lymphoid tissue. In: Ader R, Felten DL, Cohen N, editors. Psychoneuroimmunology. San Diego (CA): Academic Press; 1991. p. 87–101.

39. Irwin MR, Miller AH. Depressive disorders and immunity: 20 years of progress and discovery. Brain Behav Immun 2007;21(4):374–83.

40. Elenkov IJ, Wilder RL, Chrousos GP, et al. The sympathetic nerve–an integrative interface between two supersystems: the brain and the immune system. Pharmacol Rev 2000;52(4):595–638.

41. Chrousos GP. Stress and disorders of the stress system. Nat Rev Endocrinol 2009;5(7):374–81.

42. Khan MM, Sansoni P, Silverman ED, et al. Beta-adrenergic receptors on human suppressor, helper, and cytolytic lymphocytes. Biochem Pharmacol 1986;35(7):1137–42.

43. Hellstrand K, Hermodsson S, Strannegard O. Evidence for beta-adrenoceptor-mediated regulation of human natural killer cells. J Immunol 1985;134(6):4095–9.

44. Zorilla EP, Luborsky L, McKay JR. The relationship of depression and stressors to immunological assays: a meta-analytic review. Brain Behav Immun 2001;15(3):199–226.

45. Kiecolt-Glaser JK, McGuire L, Robles TF, et al. Emotions, morbidity, and mortality: new perspectives from psychoneuroimmunology. Annu Rev Psychol 2002;53:83–107.

46. Dunn GP, Bruce AT, Ikeda H, et al. Cancer immunoediting: from immunosurveillance to tumor escape. Nat Immunol 2002;3(11):991–8.

47. Cerwenka A, Lanier L. Natural killer cells, viruses and cancer. Nat Rev Immunol 2001;1(1):41–9.

48. Reiche EM, Nunes SO, Morimoto HK. Stress, depression, the immune system, and cancer. Lancet Oncol 2004;5(10):617–25.

49. Kiecolt-Glaser JK, Robles TF, Heffner KL, et al. Psycho-oncology and cancer: psychoneuroimmunology and cancer. Ann Oncol 2002;13(Suppl 4):165–9.

50. Heffner KL, Loving TJ, Robles TF, et al. Examining psychosocial factors related to cancer incidence and progression: in search of the silver lining. Brain Behav Immun 2003;17(Suppl 1):S109–11.

51. Saul AN, Oberyszyn TM, Daugherty C, et al. Chronic stress and susceptibility to skin cancer. J Natl Cancer Inst 2005;97(23):1760–7.

52. Ben-Eliyahu S, Page GG, Yimira R, et al. Evidence that stress and surgical interventions promote tumor development by suppressing natural killer cell activity. Int J Cancer 1999;80(6):880–8.

53. Ben-Eliyahu S, Yirmiya R, Liebeskind JC, et al. Stress increases metastatic spread of a mammary tumor in rats: evidence for mediation by the immune system. Brain Behav Immun 1991;5(2):193–205.

54. Greenfeld K, Avraham R, Benish M, et al. Immune suppression while awaiting surgery and following it: dissociations between plasma cytokine levels, their induced production, and NK cell cytotoxicity. Brain Behav Immun 2007;21(4):503–13.

55. Ben-Eliyahu S. The promotion of tumor metastasis by surgery and stress: Immunological basis and implications for psychoneuroimmunology. Brain Behav Immun 2003;17:27–36.

56. Ben-Eliyahu S, Shakhar G, Page GG, et al. Suppression of NK cell activity and of resistance to metastasis by stress: a role for adrenal catecholamines and beta-adrenoceptors. Neuroimmunomodulation 2000;8(3):154–64.

57. Page GG, Ben-Eliyahu S. A role for NK cells in greater susceptibility of young rats to metastatic formation. Dev Comp Immunol 1999;23(1):87–96.

58. Levy S, Herberman R, Lippman M, et al. Correlation of stress factors with sustained depression of natural killer cell activity and predicted prognosis in patients with breast cancer. J Clin Oncol 1987;5(3):348–53.

59. Levy SM, Heberman RB, Maluish AM, et al. Prognostic risk assessment in primary breast cancer by behavioral and immunological parameters. Health Psychol 1985;4(2):99–113.

60. Levy SM, Heberman RB, Whiteside T, et al. Perceived social support and tumor estrogen/progesterone receptor status as predictors of natural killer cell activity in breast cancer patients. Psychosom Med 1990;52(1):73–85.

61. Levy SM, Herberman RB, Lee J, et al. Estrogen receptor concentration and social factors as predictors of natural killer cell activity in early-stage breast cancer patients. Confirmation of a model. Nat Immun Cell Growth Regul 1990; 9(5):313–24.

62. Levy SM, Heberman RB, Lippman M, et al. Immunological and psychosocial predictors of disease recurrence in patients with early-stage breast cancer. Behav Med 1991;17(2):67–75.

63. Varker KA, Terrell CE, Welt M, et al. Impaired natural killer cell lysis in breast cancer patients with high levels of psychological stress is associated with altered expression of killer immunoglobin-like receptors. J Surg Res 2007; 139(1):36–44.

64. Thornton LM, Andersen BL, Crespin TR, et al. Individual trajectories in stress covary with immunity during recovery from cancer diagnosis and treatments. Brain Behav Immun 2007;21(2):185–94.

65. Garland MR, Lavelle E, Doherty D, et al. Cortisol does not mediate the suppressive effects of psychiatric morbidity on natural killer cell activity: a cross-sectional study of patients with early breast cancer. Psychol Med 2004;34(3):481–90.

66. Tjemsland T, Soreide JA, Matre R, et al. Preoperative psychological variables predict immunological status in patients with operable breast cancer. Psychoon-cology 1997;6(4):311–20.

67. Von Ah D, Kang D, Carpenter J. Stress, optimism, and social support: Impact on immune responses in breast cancer. Res Nurs Health 2007;30(1):72–83.

68. McGregor BA, Antoni MH, Boyers A, et al. Cognitive-behavioral stress manage-ment increased benefit finding and immune function among women with early-stage breast cancer. J Psychosom Res 2004;56(1):1–8.

69. Blomberg BB, Alvarez JP, Diaz A, et al. Psychosocial adaptation and cellular immunity in breast cancer patients in the weeks after surgery: an exploratory study. J Psychosom Res 2009;67(5):369–76.

70. Nan K, Wei Y, Zhou FL, et al. Effects of depression on parameters of cell-medi-ated immunity in patients with digestive tract cancers. World J Gastroenterol 2004;10(2):268–72.

71. Dunigan JT, Carr BI, Steel JL. Posttraumatic growth, immunity and survival in patients with hepatoma. Dig Dis Sci 2007;52(9):2452–9.

72. Penedo FJ, Dahn JR, Kinsinger D, et al. Anger suppression mediates the rela-tionship between optimism and natural killer cell cytotoxicity in men treated for localized prostate cancer. J Psychosom Res 2006;60(4):423–7.

73. Zhou FL, Zhang WG, Wei YC, et al. Impact of comorbid anxiety and depression on quality of life and cellular immunity changes in patients with digestive tract cancers. World J Gastroenterol 2005;11(15):2313–8.

74. Lutgendorf SK, Sood AK, Andersen B, et al. Social support, psychological distress, and natural killer cell activity in ovarian cancer. J Clin Oncol 2005;23(28):7105–13.

75. Yermal SJ, Witek-Janusek L, Peterson J, et al. Perioperative pain, psychological distress, and immune function in men undergoing prostatectomy for cancer of the prostate. Biol Res Nurs 2009;11:351–62.

76. Lamkin DM, Lutgendorf SK, McGinn S, et al. Positive psychosocial factors and NKT cells in ovarian cancer patients. Brain Behav Immun 2008;22(1):65–73.

77. Lutgendorf SK, Lamkin DM, DeGeest K, et al. Depressed and anxious mood and T-cell cytokine expressing populations in ovarian cancer patients. Brain Be-hav Immun 2008;22(6):890–900.

78. Fidler IJ. Critical factors in the biology of human cancer metastasis. Am Surg 1995;61(12):1065–6.

79. Fidler IJ. Modulation of the organ microenvironment for treatment of cancer metastasis. J Natl Cancer Inst 1995;87(21):1588–92.

80. Szlosarek P, Charles KA, Balkwill FR. Tumour necrosis factor-alpha as a tumour promoter. Eur J Cancer 2006;42(6):745–50.

81. Hanahan D, Weinberg RA. The hallmarks of cancer. Cell 2000;100(1):57–70.

82. Skobe M, Fusenig NE. Tumorigenic conversion of immortal human keratinocytres through stromal cell activation. Proc Natl Acad Sci U S A 1998;95(3):1050–5.

83. Coussens LM, Werb Z. Inflammation and cancer. Nature 2002;420(6917):860–7.

84. Folkman J. Tumor angiogenesis. The molecular basis of cancer. Philadelphia: WB Saunders; 1995. p. 206–32.

85. Folkman J. What is the evidence that tumors are angiogenesis dependant? J Natl Cancer Inst 1990;82:4–6.

86. Folkman J, Klagsbrun M. Angiogenic factors. Science 1987;235(4787):442–7.

87. Fidler IJ. Molecular biology of cancer: invasion and metastasis. In: DeVita VT, Hellman S, Rosenberg S, editors. Cancer: principles and practice of oncology. 5th edition. Philadelphia: JB Lippincott; 1997. p. 135–52.

88. Sood AK, Coffin JE, Schneider GB, et al. Biological significance of focal adhesion kinase in ovarian cancer: role in migration and invasion. Am J Pathol 2004; 165(4):1087–95.
89. Sood AK, Bhatty R, Kamat AA, et al. Stress hormone mediated invasion of ovarian cancer cells. Clin Cancer Res 2006;12(2):369–75.
90. Sood A, Lutgendorf S, Cole S. Neuroendocrine regulation of cancer progression: I. Biological mechanisms and clinical relevance. In: Ader R, Cohen N, Felten D, editors, Psychoneuroimmunology, vol. IV. San Diego (CA): Elsevier; 2007. p. 233–50.
91. Thaker P, Han LY, Kamat AA, et al. Chronic stress promotes tumor growth and angiogenesis in a mouse model of ovarian carcinoma. Nat Med 2006;12(8): 939–44.
92. Sood AK, Armaiz-Pena G, Halder J, et al. Adrenergic modulation of focal adhesion kinase protects human ovarian cancer cells from anoikis. J Clin Invest 2010; 120(5):1515–23.
93. Yang EV, Kim SJ, Donovan EL, et al. Norepinephrine upregulates VEGF, IL-8, and IL-6 expression in human melanoma tumor cell lines: implications for stress-related enhancement of tumor progression. Brain Behav Immun 2009; 23(2):267–75.
94. Yang EV, Sood AK, Chen M, et al. Norepinephrine up-regulates the expression of vascular endothelial growth factor, matrix metalloproteinase (MMP)-2, and MMP-9 in nasopharyngeal carcinoma tumor cells. Cancer Res 2006;66(21): 10357–64.
95. Nilsson MB, Armaiz-Pena G, Takahashi R, et al. Stress hormones regulate IL-6 expression by human ovarian carcinoma cells through a SRC-dependent mechanism. J Biol Chem 2007;282(41):29919–26.
96. Lutgendorf SK, Lamkin DM, Jennings NB, et al. Biobehavioral influences on matrix metalloproteinase expression in ovarian carcinoma. Clin Cancer Res 2008;14(21):6839–46.
97. Lutgendorf SK, Cole S, Costanzo E, et al. Stress-related mediators stimulate vascular endothelial growth factor secretion by two ovarian cancer cell lines. Clin Cancer Res 2003;9(12):4514–21.
98. Lee J, Shahzad MM, Lin YG, et al. Surgical stress promotes tumor growth in ovarian carcinoma. Clin Cancer Res 2009;15(8):2695–702.
99. Lutgendorf SK, Johnsen EL, Cooper B, et al. Vascular endothelial growth factor and social support in patients with ovarian carcinoma. Cancer 2002;95(4): 808–15.
100. Nilsson MB, Langley RR, Fidler IJ. Interleukin-6, secreted by human ovarian carcinoma cells, is a potent proangiogenic cytokine. Cancer Res 2005;65(23): 10794–800.
101. Cohen T, Nahari D, Cerem LW, et al. Interleukin 6 induces the expression of vascular endothelial growth factor. J Biol Chem 1996;271(2):736–41.
102. Eustace D, Han X, Gooding R, et al. Interleukin 6 (IL-6) functions as an autocrine growth factor in cervical carcinomas in vitro. Gynecol Oncol 1993;50(1):15–9.
103. Obata NH, Tamakoshi K, Shibata K, et al. Effects of interleukin-6 on in vitro cell attachment, migration, and invasion of human ovarian carcinoma. Anticancer Res 1997;17(1A):337–42.
104. Kitamura Y, Morita I, Nihel Z, et al. Effects of IL-6 on tumor cells invasion of vascular endothelial monolayers. Jpn J Surg 1997;27:534–41.
105. Berek JS, Chung C, Kaldi K, et al. Serum interleukin-6 levels correlate with disease status in patients with epithelial ovarian cancer. Am J Obstet Gynecol 1991;164(4):1038–43.

106. Chopra V, Dinh TV, Hannigan E. Circulating serum levels of cytokines and angiogenic factors in patients with cervical cancer. Cancer Invest 1998; 16(3):152–9.

107. Scambia G, Testa U, Benedetti P, et al. Prognostic significance of IL-6 serum levels in patients with ovarian cancer. Br J Cancer 1995;71(2):352–6.

108. Mastorakos G, Chrousos GP, Weber JS. Recombinant interleukin-6 activates the hypothalamic pituitary adrenal axis in humans. J Clin Endocrinol Metab 1993; 77(6):1690–4.

109. Zhou D, Kusnecov A, Shurin M, et al. Exposure to physical and psychological stressors elevates plasma interleukin-6: relationship to the activation of hypothalamic-pituitary-adrenal axis. Endocrinology 1993;133(6):2523–30.

110. Spangelo BL, MacLeod RM, Isakson PC. Production of interleukin-6 by anterior pituitary cells in vitro. Endocrinology 1990;126(1):582–6.

111. Papanicolaou D, Petrides J, Tsigos C, et al. Exercise stimulates interleukin-6 secretion: inhibition by glucocorticoids and correlation with catecholamines. Am J Physiol 1996;271(3 PT 1):e601–5.

112. DeRijk R, Sternberg E. Corticosteroid action and neuroendocrine-immune interactions. Ann N Y Acad Sci 1994;746:33–41.

113. Frommberger UH, Bauer J, Haselbauer P, et al. Interleukin-6 plasma levels in depression and schizophrenia: comparison between the acute state and after remission. Eur Arch Psychiatry Clin Neurosci 1997;247(4):228–33.

114. Lutgendorf S, Garand L, Buckwalter K, et al. Life stress, mood disturbance, and elevated IL-6 in healthy older women. J Gerontol A Biol Sci Med Sci 1999;54(9): M434–9.

115. Maes M, Bosmans E, de Jongh R, et al. Increased serum IL-6 and IL-1 receptor antagonist concentrations in major depression and treatment resistant depression. Cytokine 1997;9(11):853–8.

116. Krause A, Holtmann H, Eickemeier S, et al. Stress-activated protein kinase/Jun N-terminal kinase is required for interleukin (IL)-1 induced IL-6 and IL-8 gene expression in the human epidermal carcinoma cell line KB. J Biol Chem 1998; 273(37):23681–9.

117. Costanzo ES, Lutgendorf SK, Sood AK, et al. Psychosocial factors and interleukin-6 among women with advanced ovarian cancer. Cancer 2005;104(2): 305–13.

118. Suzuki K, Yamada M, Kurakake S, et al. Circulating cytokines and hormones with immunosuppressive but neutrophil-priming potentials rise after endurance exercise in humans. Eur J Appl Physiol 2000;81(4):281–7.

119. Tayama E, Hayashida M, Oda T, et al. Recovery from lymphocytopenia following extracorporeal circulation: simple indicator to assess surgical stress. Artif Organs 1999;23(8):736–40.

120. Landen CN, Lin YG, Armaiz-Pena GN, et al. Neuroendocrine modulation of signal transducer and activator of transcription-3 in ovarian cancer. Cancer Res 2007;67(21):10389–96.

121. Masur K, Niggemann B, Zanker KS, et al. Norepinephrine-induced migration of SW 480 colon carcinoma cells is inhibited by beta-blockers. Cancer Res 2001; 61(7):2866–9.

122. Drell TL, Joseph J, Lang K, et al. Effects of neurotransmitters on the chemokinesis and chemotaxis of MDA-MB-468 human breast carcinoma cells. Breast Cancer Res Treat 2003;80:63–70.

123. Yang E, Bane CM, MacCallum RC, et al. Stress-related modulation of matrix metalloproteinase expression. J Neuroimmunol 2002;133(1–2):144–50.

124. Lutgendorf SK, Weinrib AZ, Penedo F, et al. Interleukin-6, cortisol, and depressive symptoms in ovarian cancer patients. J Clin Oncol 2008;26(29):4820–7.

125. Lutgendorf SK, DeGeest K, Sung CY, et al. Depression, social support, and beta-adrenergic transcription control in human ovarian cancer. Brain Behav Immun 2009;23(2):176–83.

126. Balkwill F, Mantovani A. Inflammation and cancer: back to Virchow? Lancet 2001;357(9255):539–45.

127. Pollard JW. Tumour-educated macrophages promote tumour progression and metastasis. Nat Rev Cancer 2004;4(1):71–8.

128. Sica A, Schioppa T, Mantovani A, et al. Tumour-associated macrophages are a distinct M2 polarised population promoting tumour. Eur J Cancer 2006; 42(6):717–27.

129. Huang S, Van Arsdall M, Tedjarati S, et al. Contributions of stromal metalloproteinase-9 to angiogenesis and growth of human ovarian carcinoma in mice. J Natl Cancer Inst 2002;94(15):1134–42.

130. Hagemann T, Robinson SC, Schulz M, et al. Enhanced invasiveness of breast cancer cell lines upon co-cultivation with macrophages is due to TNF-alpha dependent up-regulation of matrix metalloproteases. Carcinogenesis 2004; 25(8):1543–9.

131. Sica A, Allavena P, Mantovani A. Cancer related inflammation: the macrophage connection. Cancer Lett 2008;267(2):204–15.

132. Bingle L, Brown NJ, Lewis CE. The role of tumour-associated macrophages in tumour progression: implications for new anticancer therapies. J Pathol 2002; 196(3):254–65.

133. Balkwill F, Charles KA, Mantovani A. Smoldering and polarized inflammation in the initiation and promotion of malignant disease. Cancer Cell 2005;7(3):211–7.

134. Tsutsui S, Yasuda K, Suzuki K, et al. Macrophage infiltration and its prognostic implications in breast cancer: the relationship with VEGF expression and microvessel density. Oncol Rep 2005;14(2):425–31.

135. Miller GE, Cohen S, Ritchey AK. Chronic psychological stress and the regulation of pro-inflammatory cytokines: a glucocorticoid-resistance model. Health Psychol 2002;21(6):531–41.

136. Black PH. Stress and the inflammatory response: a review of neurogenic inflammation. Brain Behav Immun 2002;16(6):622–53.

137. Szelenyi J, Kiss JP, Puskas E, et al. Contribution of differently localized alpha 2- and beta-adrenoceptors in the modulation of TNF-alpha and IL-10 production in endotoxemic mice. Ann N Y Acad Sci 2000;917:145–53.

138. Van Miert A. Present concepts on the inflammatory modulators with special reference to cytokines. Vet Res Commun 2002;26(2):111–26.

139. Elenkov IJ, Chrousos GP. Stress hormones, proinflammatory and antiinflammatory cytokines, and autoimmunity. Ann N Y Acad Sci 2002;966:290–303.

140. Cole SW, Hawkley LC, Arevalo JM, et al. Social regulation of gene expression in human leukocytes. Genome Biol 2007;8(9):R189.

141. Raison CL, Miller AH. When not enough is too much: the role of insufficient glucocorticoid signaling in the pathophysiology of stress-related disorders. Am J Psychiatry 2003;160(9):1554–65.

142. Maier S, Watkins L. Cytokines for psychologists: implications of bidirectional immune to brain communication for understanding behavior, mood, and cognition. Psychol Rev 1998;105(1):83–107.

143. Raison CL, Capuron L, Miller AH. Cytokines sing the blues: inflammation and the pathogenesis of depression. Trends Immunol 2006;27(1):24–31.

144. Capuron L, Dantzer R. Cytokines and depression: the need for a new paradigm. Brain Behav Immun 2003;17:S119–24.

145. Miller GE, Chen E, Sze J, et al. A functional genomic fingerprint of chronic stress in humans: blunted glucocorticoid and increased NF-kappaB signaling. Biol Psychiatry 2008;64(4):266–72.

146. Spiegel D, Giese-Davis J. Depression and cancer: mechanisms and disease progression. Biol Psychiatry 2003;54(3):269–82.

147. Musselman DL, Miller AH, Porter MR, et al. Higher than normal plasma inter-leukin-6 concentrations in cancer patients with depression: preliminary findings. Am J Psychiatry 2001;158(8):1252–7.

148. Jehn CF, Kuehnhardt D, Bartholomae A, et al. Biomarkers of depression in cancer patients. Cancer 2006;107(11):2723–9.

149. Rich T, Innominato PF, Boerner J, et al. Elevated serum cytokines correlated with altered behavior, serum cortisol rhythm, and dampened 24-hour rest-activity patterns in patients with metastatic colorectal cancer. Clin Cancer Res 2005; 11(5):1757–64.

150. Weinrib A, Sephton SE, DeGeest K, et al. Diurnal cortisol dysregulation: links with depression and functional disability in women with ovarian cancer. Cancer 2010;116(18):4410–9.

151. Bower JE, Ganz PA, Aziz N, et al. Fatigue and proinflammatory cytokine activity in breast cancer survivors. Psychosom Med 2002;64(4):604–11.

152. Collado-Hidalgo A, Bower ME, Ganz PA, et al. Inflammatory biomarkers for persistent fatigue in breast cancer survivors. Clin Cancer Res 2006;12(9):2759–66.

153. Bower JE, Ganz PA, Dickerson SS, et al. Diurnal cortisol rhythm and fatigue in breast cancer survivors. Psychoneuroendocrinology 2005;30(1):92–100.

154. Collado-Hidalgo A, Bower JE, Ganz PA, et al. Cytokine gene polymorphisms and fatigue in breast cancer survivors: early findings. J Brain Behav Immun 2008;22(8):1197–200.

155. Jacobsen PB, Jim HS. Psychosocial interventions for anxiety and depression in adult cancer patients: achievements and challenges. CA Cancer J Clin 2008; 58(4):214–30.

156. Uitterhoeve RJ, Vernooy M, Litjens M, et al. Psychosocial interventions for patients with advanced cancer - a systematic review of the literature. Br J Cancer 2004;91(6):1050–62.

157. Daniels J, Kissane DW. Psychosocial interventions for cancer patients. Curr Opin Oncol 2008;20(4):367–71.

158. Antoni MH, Lechner SC, Kazi A, et al. How stress management improves quality of life after treatment for breast cancer. J Consult Clin Psychol 2006;74(6):1143–52.

159. Spiegel D, Bloom G, Kramer J, et al. Effect of psychosocial treatment on survival of patients with metastatic breast cancer. Lancet 1989;2(8668):888–91.

160. Fawzy FI, Fawzy NW, Hyun CS, et al. Malignant melanoma: effects of an early structured psychiatric intervention, coping, and affective state on recurrence and survival 6 years later. Arch Gen Psychiatry 1993;50(9):681–9.

161. Fox BA. A hypothesis about Spiegel et al.'s 1989 paper on psychosocial intervention and breast cancer survival. Psychooncology 1998;7(5):361–70.

162. Kogon MM, Biswas A, Pearl D, et al. Effects of medical and psychotherapeutic treatment on the survival of women with metastatic breast carcinoma. Cancer 1997;80(2):225–30.

163. Coyne J, Stefanek M, Palmer S. Psychotherapy and survival in cancer: the conflict between hope and evidence. Psychol Bull 2007;133(3):367–94.

164. Cunningham LL, Andrykowski MA, Wilson JF, et al. Physical symptoms, distress, and breast cancer risk perceptions in women with benign breast problems. Health Psychol 1998;17(4):371–5.

165. Edelman S, Bell DR, Kidman AD. A group cognitive behavioral therapy programme with metastatic breast cancer patients. Psychooncology 1999;8(4):295–305.

166. Edelman S, Lemon J, Bell DR, et al. Effects of group CBT on the survival time of patients with metastatic breast cancer. Psychooncology 1999;8(6):474–81.

167. Goodwin P, Leszcz M, Ennis M, et al. The effect of group psychosocial support on survival in metastatic breast cancer. N Engl J Med 2001; 345(24):1719–26.

168. Kissane DW, Grabsch B, Clarke DM, et al. Supportive-expressive group therapy for women with metastatic breast cancer: survival and psychosocial outcome from a randomized controlled trial. Psychooncology 2007;16(4):277–86.

169. Spiegel D, Butler LD, Giese-Davis J, et al. Effects of supportive-expressive group therapy on survival of patients with metastatic breast cancer: a randomized prospective trial. Cancer 2007;110(5):1130–7.

170. Ilnyckyj A, Farber J, Cheang M, et al. A randomized controlled trial of psychotherapeutic intervention in cancer patients. Ann R Coll Physicians Surg Can 1994;27:93–6.

171. Gellert GA, Maxwell RM, Siegel BS. Survival of breast cancer patients receiving adjunctive psychosocial support therapy: a 10-year follow-up study. J Clin Oncol 1993;11(1):66–9.

172. Kissane DW, Love A, Hatton H, et al. Effect of cognitive-existential group therapy on survival in early-stage breast cancer. J Clin Oncol 2004;22(21):4255–60.

173. Andersen BL, Yang HC, Farrar WB, et al. Psychologic intervention improves survival for breast cancer patients: a randomized clinical trial. Cancer 2008; 113(12):3450–8.

174. Kuchler T, Bestmann B, Rappat S, et al. Impact of psychotherapeutic support for patients with gastrointestinal cancer undergoing surgery: 10-year survival results of a randomized trial. J Clin Oncol 2007;25(19):2702–8.

175. Kuchler T, Henne-Bruns D, Rappat S, et al. Impact of psychotherapeutic support on gastrointestinal cancer patients undergoing surgery: survival results of a trial. Hepatogastroenterology 1999;46(25):322–35.

176. Fawzy FI, Canada AL, Fawzy NW. Malignant melanoma: effects of a brief, structured psychiatric intervention on survival and recurrence at 10-year follow-up. Arch Gen Psychiatry 2003;60(1):100–3.

177. Phillips KM, Antoni MH, Lechner SC, et al. Stress management intervention reduces serum cortisol and increases relaxation during treatment for nonmetastatic breast cancer. Psychosom Med 2008;70(9):1044–9.

178. Antoni MH, Wimberly SR, Lechner SC, et al. Reduction of cancer-specific thought intrusions and anxiety symptoms with a stress management intervention among women undergoing treatment for breast cancer. Am J Psychiatry 2006; 163(10):1791–7.

179. Antoni MH, Lechner S, Diaz A, et al. Cognitive behavioral stress management effects on psychosocial and physiological adaptation in women undergoing treatment for breast cancer. Brain Behav Immun 2009;23(5):580–91.

180. Andersen BL, Farrar WB, Golden-Kreutz DM, et al. Psychological, behavioral, and immune changes after a psychological intervention: a clinical trial. J Clin Oncol 2004;22(17):3570–80.

181. Andersen BL, Farrar WB, Golden-Kreutz D, et al. Distress reduction from a psychological intervention contributes to improved health for cancer patients. Brain Behav Immun 2007;21(7):953–61.

182. Thornton LM, Andersen BL, Schuler TA, et al. A psychological intervention reduces inflammatory markers by alleviating depressive symptoms: secondary analysis of a randomized controlled trial. Psychosom Med 2009; 71(7):715–24.

183. Carlson LE, Garland SN. Impact of mindfulness-based stress reduction (MBSR) on sleep, mood, stress and fatigue symptoms in cancer outpatients. Int J Behav Med 2005;12(4):278–85.

184. Carlson LE, Speca M, Faris P, et al. One year pre-post intervention follow-up of psychological, immune, endocrine and blood pressure outcomes of mindfulness-based stress reduction (MBSR) in breast and prostate cancer outpatients. Brain Behav Immun 2007;21(8):1038–49.

185. Carlson LE, Speca M, Patel KD, et al. Mindfulness-based stress reduction in relation to quality of life, mood, symptoms of stress, and immune parameters in breast and prostate cancer outpatients. Psychosom Med 2003;65(4): 571–81.

186. Witek-Janusek L, Albuquerque K, Chroniak KR, et al. Effect of mindfulness based stress reduction on immune function, quality of life and coping in women newly diagnosed with early stage breast cancer. Brain Behav Immun 2008; 22(6):969–81.

187. Eremin O, Walker MB, Simpson E, et al. Immuno-modulatory effects of relaxation training and guided imagery in women with locally advanced breast cancer undergoing multimodality therapy: a randomized controlled trial. Breast 2009; 18(1):17–25.

188. Gruber BL, Hersh SP, Hall NRS, et al. Immunological responses of breast cancer patients to behavioral interventions. Biofeedback Self Regul 1993;18(1):1–22.

189. Lengacher CA, Bennett MP, Gonzalez L, et al. Immune responses to guided imagery during breast cancer treatment. Biol Res Nurs 2008;9(3):205–14.

190. Bakke AC, Purtzer MZ, Newton P. The effect of hypnotic-guided imagery on psychological well-being and immune function in patients with prior breast cancer. J Psychosom Res 2002;53(6):1131–7.

191. Schedlowski M, Jung C, Schimanski G, et al. Effects of behavioral intervention on plasma cortisol and lymphocytes in breast cancer patients: an exploratory study. Psychooncology 1994;3:181–7.

192. Savard J, Simard S, Giguere I, et al. Randomized clinical trial on cognitive therapy for depression in women with metastatic breast cancer: psychological and immunological effects. Palliat Support Care 2006;4(3):219–37.

193. Ross L, Frederiksen K, Boesen SH, et al. No effect on survival of home psychosocial intervention in a randomized study of Danish colorectal cancer patients. Psychooncology 2009;18(8):875–85.

194. Hosaka T, Tokuda Y, Sugiyama Y, et al. Effects of a structured psychiatric intervention on immune function of cancer patients. Tokai J Exp Clin Med 2000; 25(4–6):183–8.

195. Savard J, Simard S, Ivers H, et al. Randomized study on the efficacy of cognitive-behavioral therapy for insomnia secondary to breast cancer, part II: immunologic effects. J Clin Oncol 2005;23(25):6097–106.

196. Eismann EA, Lush E, Sephton SE. Circadian effects in cancer-relevant psychoneuroendocrine and immune pathways. Psychoneuroendocrinology 2010;35(7): 963–76.

197. Sephton S, Spiegel D. Circadian disruption in cancer: a neuroendocrine-immune pathway from stress to disease? Brain Behav Immun 2003;17(5):321–8.
198. Capuron L, Gumnick JF, Musselman DL, et al. Neurobehavioral effects of interferon-alpha in cancer patients: phenomenology and paroxetine responsiveness of symptom dimensions. Neuropsychopharmacology 2002;26(5):643–52.
199. Morrow GR, Hickok JT, Roscoe JA, et al. Differential effects of paroxetine on fatigue and depression: a randomized, double-blind trial from the University of Rochester Cancer Center Community Clinical Oncology Program. J Clin Oncol 2003;21(24):4635–41.
200. Kubera M, Grygier B, Arteta B, et al. Age-dependent stimulatory effect of desipramine and fluoxetine pretreatment on metastasis formation by B16F10 melanoma in male C57BL/6 mice. Pharmacol Rep 2009;61:1113–26.
201. Lee CS, Kim YJ, Jang ER, et al. Fluoxetine induces apoptosis in ovarian carcinoma cell line OVCAR-3 through reactive oxygen species-dependent activation of nuclear factor-kB. Basic Clin Pharmacol Toxicol 2010;106(6):446–53.
202. Melemed AS, Mockbee C, Orlando M. Comprehensive review of chemotherapy in patients with metastatic breast cancer. J Clin Oncol 2005;23(31):8139–40.
203. Ben-Eliyahu S, Page GG, Schleifer SJ. Stress, NK cells, and cancer: still a promissory note. Brain Behav Immun 2007;21(7):881–7.
204. Perron L, Bairati I, Harel F, et al. Antihypertensive drug use and the risk of prostate cancer. Cancer Causes Control 2004;15:535–41.
205. Avraham R, Benish M, Inbar S, et al. Synergism between immunostimulation and prevention of surgery-induced immune suppression: an approach to reduce post-operative tumor progression. Brain Behav Immun 2010;24(6):952–8.
206. Shakhar G, Ben-Eliyahu S. Potential prophylactic measures against postoperative immunosuppression: could they reduce recurrence rates in oncological patients? Ann Clin Oncol 2003;10(8):972–92.
207. Uchida A, Kariya Y, Okamoto N, et al. Prediction of postoperative clinical course by autologous tumor-killing activity in lung cancer patients. J Natl Cancer Inst 1990;82(21):1697–701.
208. Mccoy JL, Rucker R, Petros JA. Cell-mediated immunity to tumor-associated antigens is a better predictor of survival in early stage breast cancer than stage, grade or lymph node status. Breast Cancer Res Treat 2000;60(3):227–34.
209. Bacigalupo A. Results of allogeneic hematopoietic stem cell transplantation for hematologic malignancies. In: Hoffman R, editor. Hematology: basic principles and practice. 4th edition. Philadelphia: Churchill Livingstone; 2005. p. 1713–26.
210. Schriber JR, Forman SJ. Autologous transplantation for hematologic malignancies and solid tumors. In: Hoffman R, editor. Hematology: basic principles and practice. 4th edition. Philadelphia: Churchill Livingstone; 2005. p. 1727–38.
211. Porrata LF, Litzow M, Markovic SN. Immune reconstitution after autologous hematopoietic stem cell transplantation. Mayo Clin Proc 2001;76(4):407–12.
212. Neitzert CS, Ritvo P, Dancey J, et al. The psychosocial impact of bone marrow transplantation: a review of the literature. Bone Marrow Transplant 1998;22(5):409–22.
213. Colon EA, Callies AL, Popkin MK, et al. Depressed mood and other variables related to bone marrow transplantation survival in acute leukemia. Psychosomatics 1991;32(4):420–5.
214. Molassiotis A, Van den Akker OBA, Milligan DW, et al. Symptom distress, coping style and biological variables as predictors of survival after bone marrow transplantation. J Psychosom Res 1997;42(3):275–85.

215. Hoodin F, Kalbfleisch KR, Thornton J, et al. Psychosocial influences on 305 adults' survival after bone marrow transplantation; depression, smoking, and behavioral self-regulation. J Psychosom Res 2004;57(2):145–54.
216. Rodrigue JR, Pearman TP, Moreb J. Morbidity and mortality following bone marrow transplantation: predictive utility of pre-BMT affective functioning, compliance, and social support stability. Int J Behav Med 1999;6(3):241–54.
217. Porrata LF, Markovic SN. Timely reconstitution of immune competence affects clinical outcome following autologous stem cell transplantation. Clin Exp Med 2004;4(2):78–85.
218. Peggs KS, Mackinnon S. Immune reconstitution following haematopoietic stem cell transplantation. Br J Haematol 2004;124(4):407–20.
219. Auletta JJ, Lazarus HM. Immune restoration following hematopoietic stem cell transplantation: an evolving target. Bone Marrow Transplant 2005;35(9):835–7.

The Adverse Effects of Psychological Stress on Immunoregulatory Balance: Applications to Human Inflammatory Diseases

Gailen D. Marshall Jr, MD, PhD

KEYWORDS

- Stress • Immunoregulation • Single nucleotide polymorphisms
- Inflammation

Psychoneuroimmunology (PNI) research has long been concerned with the relationships between excessive psychological stress and health risks. Ancient medical authorities recognized the relationships between stress and health,[1] and the negative impact on inflammatory processes was the presumed basis for the increased incidence of infections seen in high-stress populations.[2] Only recently have the medical and scientific communities come to appreciate that psychological stress cannot only increase susceptibility to infection but also impair wound healing and enhance hypersensitivity inflammatory states, such as allergy, asthma, and various autoimmune conditions.[3]

Two great pioneers of PNI research, Ader and Cohen, began their work when the technology of immunology research was in its relative infancy. Accordingly, the idea that stress was largely immunosuppressive prevailed as most of the animal models were designed to show increased susceptibility to infection with exposure to specific stressors. Yet there emerged an interest, beginning in the older medical literature, that described relationships linking stress with various inflammatory diseases.[4]

Supported in part by grants 1 CPI MP061018-02, 5 R21 AT002938-02, and 1 R21 HL96086-01 from the National Institutes of Health and the Health Resources and Services Administration, Department of Health and Human Services.

Laboratory of Behavioral Immunology Research, Division of Clinical Immunology and Allergy, Department of Medicine, The University of Mississippi Medical Center, 2500 North State Street N416, Jackson, MS 39216-4505, USA

E-mail address: gmarshall@umc.edu

As technology for more accurately and definitively assessing various components of the immune response has developed, research has confirmed that high levels of psychological stress have effects far beyond merely suppressing immune function, including altering immunoregulatory networks and causing increased risk for allergic and autoimmune diseases in both young and older individuals. In the past 30 years, PNI research has established that the brain and the immune system are inextricably linked through a variety of pathways that include the hypophyseal-pituitary-adrenal axis and other endocrine organs, including the thyroid, gonadal, and adrenomedullary, as well as autonomic nervous system components.[5] Although their neuroendocrine pathways are not identical, both anxiety and depression are associated with similar effects on regulatory and effector immune components.[6] This association has been confirmed through several observational studies; people with inflammatory diseases, such as asthma and autoimmunity, have increased prevalence of anxiety and depressive states.[7] Additionally, people with anxiety and depressive disorders are at increased risk for various inflammatory diseases.[8]

Further research has shown that certain therapeutic agents that impact neuroendocrine or autonomic pathways can also affect how individuals respond to stress-induced changes in immune function.[9] All of these findings have been firmly established in animal models, normal human volunteers, and even some patient populations with certain inflammatory disease states. In addition, investigators have shown that demographic parameters, such as gender, race, body mass index, age, and socioeconomic status, have an impact on the prevalence and severity of conditions, such as cardiovascular disease,[10] hypertension,[11] and diabetes.[12] Individual differences based upon these demographic parameters are also likely modifiers of stress-related immune effects.

This brief review provides an overview of the major immune mechanisms reported to be most adversely affected by stress and a brief discussion of current research, and clinical and policy issues that need to be addressed to more effectively implement specific stress reduction/management strategies for individual patients with inflammatory diseases.

NORMAL IMMUNE RESPONSES

In normal humans, presentation of antigen for a specific protective immune response elicits a complex series of events that result in a mixed cellular and humoral protective response, the intensity and nature of which depends upon the specific inciting antigen.[13] Generally speaking, extracellular pathogens (ie, bacteria) incite a primarily humoral response; whereas, intracellular pathogens (eg, virus, fungi, mycobacteria) elicit a cell-mediated response. Antiviral immunity is particularly complex because both mechanisms are necessary for host resistance; cellular immunity is needed to eliminate the virus-infected host cells and humoral immunity is needed to produce antiviral-neutralizing antibodies to prevent reinfection. The host-immune response has a variety of mechanisms to direct the immune response into the humoral versus cellular direction, including the nature of antigen presenting cells, major histocompatibility complex restriction, and availability of specific T-cell and B-cell components; however, the central control of the cellular versus humoral response to an antigenic challenge appears to be via production of specific cytokines.

A central source of these cytokines comes from CD4+ helper T-cell subpopulations, often referred to as Th1 and Th2 cells.[14] Human Th1 cells secrete several different cytokines with the seminal Th1 cytokine being interferon gamma (IFNγ). These cytokines are important factors in the generation of cellular immune responses, including antigen-specific cytotoxic T lymphocytes and natural killer cells. Additionally, IFNγ in particular has an antagonistic activity against Th2 cytokines. Interleukin-12 (IL-12) and IL-18, produced primarily by activated macrophages, play a central role in upregulating IFNγ production. In contrast, Th2 cells secrete various other cytokines, including IL-4, IL-5, IL-9, IL-10, and IL-13, which are involved in isotype switching of B cells as well as proliferation and differentiation into antibody-secreting plasma cells. In particular, IL-4 and IL-13 are involved in the isotype switch from IgM to IgE, the antibody responsible for classical allergic disease. IL-4 and IL-10 are also regulatory cytokines, antagonizing the activities of Th1 cytokines.

IMMUNE DEVIATION VERSUS IMMUNE REGULATION

In the normal host response, as previously described above, specificity, intensity, and duration are all essential components of normal host immunity. When any or all of these components become dysfunctional, immune-based diseases can be expected to develop, at least in susceptible patients. Normal regulatory mechanisms are designed to keep type, duration, and intensity of immune responses within normal homeostatic boundaries. Specificity involves both epitope recognition on a molecular level and host defense against intracellular versus extracellular pathogens on an organismic level. The pathogen discrimination is called *immune deviation* and is mediated by Th1 (for intracellular pathogen defense) and Th2 cytokines (for extracellular pathogen defense). Additionally, the intensity and duration of these responses must also be regulated. Recent studies have indicated the presence of T-cell subpopulations that can regulate intensity and duration of various immune responses. Various names have been used to describe these cells, including suppressor T cells, Th3 cells, Tr1 cells, and, most recently, regulatory T cells (T_{REG}). There appear to be at least 2 types of CD4+ T_{REGS} in normal humans characterized by their surface markers CD4 and CD25 as well as intracellular expression of Fox P3, a DNA-binding transcription factor that is highly expressed in T_{REGS}.[15]

IMPACT OF PSYCHOLOGICAL STRESS ON IMMUNOREGULATION

Stress is best thought of as a psychophysiological process, usually experienced as a negative emotional state, which is the appraisal of situational and psychological factors. Stressors, defined as events posing threat, harm, or challenge, are judged in the context of dispositional and environmental factors and, if appraised as menacing or challenging, produce specific responses directed at reducing the stress. A common clinical observation is the adverse relationship between stress and human disease. Indeed, various sources have estimated that up to 75% of all visits to physicians' offices are stress-related. This finding appears to be particularly true in relationship to clinical conditions characterized by immune-based dysfunctions, such as increased susceptibility to infections,[16] allergic diseases, and asthma.[17] Stress is also suspected to play a role in morbidity and mortality in other immune-based diseases, such as cancer,[18] HIV disease,[19] inflammatory bowel diseases,[20] and even immune senescence.[21] Stress may also cause persistent increases in sympathetic nervous system activity, including increased blood pressure,[22] heart rate, catecholamine secretion,[23] and platelet aggregation, which may explain, at least in part, the known association between stress, immune alterations, and cardiovascular disease.[24] Although stress-induced immune dysfunctions were once thought of primarily as immunosuppressive, more recent data have suggested that immunoregulatory dysfunctions may play a more central role in stress-induced immune alterations. Thus, because of an inappropriate, rather than deficient, immune response, otherwise healthy individuals may, at times of significant stress, have increased incidence, severity, or duration of multiple distinct conditions.[3] This increased incidence could be expected to significantly affect the performance, stamina, or durability of these individuals.

The psychological and behavioral consequences of stress may have additional, albeit indirect, effects on health by increasing incidence or severity of negative affects, increases in health-impairing behaviors (eg, poor diet, lack of exercise, substance abuse), poor sleep, and decreased quality of life.[25] These research studies suggest that stress-induced changes in psychological, behavioral, or physiologic functioning can be harmful and may result in negative health consequences through direct and indirect mechanisms. The clinical significance of these sympathetic nervous system and immune system changes must still be defined for specific patient populations. It is reasonable to conclude, however that such stress-induced inflammatory changes would adversely affect health in many individuals, particularly those with underlying inflammatory diseases.

EFFECTS OF STRESS ON IMMUNOREGULATORY BALANCE

As PNI developed, early studies suggested that psychological stress was primarily immunosuppressive in action because the models were focused on increased susceptibility to infections and decreased vaccine responses.[26] The author's group and others provided evidence that stress could alter the Th1/Th2 cytokine balance with strong deviation toward the Th2 component, which could not only increase susceptibility to certain infections but increase clinical activity of various hypersensitivity diseases.[27–29] More recent work is showing that stress, both acute and chronic, can alter the balance in fashions that may increase risk for (and thus susceptibility to) developing clinical conditions, such as asthma, coronary artery disease, or diabetes.[30]

Although there are several studies that report that chronic clinical stress and in vitro presence of stress hormones, such as corticosteroids and catecholamines, can significantly alter the Th1/Th2 balance, little has been published examining the effects of psychological stress on T_{REG} expression.[31] Of those studies that have been published, methodological differences make interpretation and conclusions difficult. Yet many of the inflammatory diseases reported to be adversely affected by stress have distinct Th1 or Th2 predominance as part of their pathophysiology.[32] What is common to many inflammatory diseases is a defect in number or function of various immunoregulatory components, which indicates a significant need for more intensive studies into the effects of stress on immunoregulatory circuits in normal hosts as well as those with inflammatory diseases. It is encouraging to observe that the body of work presented by others in this volume establishes beyond reasonable doubt that chronic (and in some instances acute) psychological stress is associated with adverse health outcomes for a variety of infectious, malignant, and inflammatory diseases.

WHICH TEST REVEALS WHICH DYSFUNCTION FOR WHICH ILLNESS?

As in all areas of biomedical research, PNI has an abundance of different instruments and methodologies that measure levels of stress and stress perception, anxiety, depression, anger, loneliness, and other emotional states that have been validated in various research settings. Similar methods exist to assess endocrine, immune, and molecular effects of experimental or naturalistic stress. The data are robust and compelling *on a population* (or subpopulation) basis. However, a major limitation to clinical utility of stress research data for assessment and treatment of individual patients is the expected variability in population data, which can significantly limit the ability to identify the most stress susceptible patients for individual, customized, therapeutic interventions.

A critical challenge for PNI researchers, in addition to continuing the excellent ongoing mechanism-based studies, is to find stable biomarkers that will allow individuals to be assigned to various categories in terms of intrinsic and situational risk. When one considers the various pathways put forth to explain the impact of psychological stress on immune function,[33] there are multiple points along the pathways for variability, from diversity in the individual perception of a given stressor to differences in levels of stress hormone production, hormone receptor expression, and density on specific immune cellular elements to disparity in numbers of immune cells, effector/regulatory ratios, cytokine receptors, and cytokine levels. Any or all of these factors, alone or in combination, may result in differing clinical consequences.

When searching for stable biomarkers, genetic approaches are often attractive because of the straightforward methodology and the relative stability of genetic biomarkers. Combined with the understanding gained from previous PNI work, searching for specific gene expression or variability in well-characterized stress models may offer opportunities to find stable biomarkers for stress responses. For example, gene microarrays can be useful as a screening tool to compare and contrast individual responses to the same stressor. Single nucleotide polymorphisms (SNP) are an increasingly popular approach to biomarker identification in disease-associational research and can also be useful in PNI studies. Categorizing subpopulation of research participants in terms of SNPs for stress hormone receptors, cytokine receptors, hormone, and cytokine promoters may hold promise for stratifying risk, particularly if taken in combination.

Other approaches to identifying biomarkers include the use of surrogate markers, that is, an assay that identifies a substance that changes with stress but is not directly involved in the mechanistic pathway. An example is α amylase analyzed in the saliva as a surrogate measure of blood catecholamine levels. The amylase is produced and secreted into the saliva as blood catecholamines (epinephrine and norepinephrine) bind to their receptors on the salivary acinar cells, activating them to produce and secrete amylase.[34] These potential biomarkers must have certain characteristics to have any significant clinical utility: (1) They should be a marker that will increase with specific stressful situations and decrease with effective resolution of the stressful situation; (2) They should be stable enough to be obtained at various times and clinical situations (hospital, outpatient clinic); (3) They should be reflective of a defined pathway affected by the stress. For example, serum IgE has been noted to be elevated in certain stressful situations.[35] Given the knowledge that IgE increases with increased IL-4 (Th2) production and stressful situations can change the Th1/Th2 balance toward Th2,[36] it is reasonable to suggest that a clinical laboratory test, such as serum IgE, could possibly have value in assessment of the clinical impact of life stressors on the underlying immune system of the host that could identify risk for inflammatory disease; and (4) Ideally, the laboratory test biomarker should correlate with the intensity and duration of the stressful experience. There are other laboratory tests that can provide chronic information in other clinical settings, such as the Hemoglobin A1C test, which correlates with overall glucose control for the previous 3 months in patients with diabetes. Such stress susceptibility tests could, at least in theory, be useful to assess the impact of chronic (or perhaps severe and/or repetitive acute) stress on host immunity.

FUTURE DIRECTIONS

PNI researchers are actively responding to the call for translational research in the field to identify specific risk factors and develop scientifically sound rationales for interventions in specific disease states as well as to provide prophylactic stress management strategies to aid in healthy aging lifestyles. We are rapidly entering the next phase of translational studies that will further define modifiers of individual stress perceptions, including cultural influences; learned behavior; socioeconomic conditions; and general healthy living behaviors, such as exercise regimens, body habitus, and use of various substances (eg, alcohol, recreational psychoactive drugs, and tobacco). Such modifiers must be accounted for when studying degrees of stress-induced immune dysfunction. The search for biomarkers that can identify stress susceptibility in individuals should focus on those that correlate well with ultimate clinical outcomes, thus allowing rapid assessment of specific interventional strategies in specific patient populations.

Although the modern mainstream Western medical community has, until recently, largely minimized or even ignored the potential effects of psychological stress as a confounder for therapeutic response or even a risk factor for immune-based inflammatory diseases, research opportunities are now abundant. Over the past decade, the field has advanced to the point where sophisticated cellular and molecular immunology techniques are being used to identify effects of stress on various components of host immunity from toll-like receptors[37] to regulatory networks involving cytokines and regulatory T cell populations.[38]

Significant challenges face researchers striving to close the knowledge gaps that currently hinder the development of effective modes of diagnosing and developing appropriate therapies for stress-exacerbated conditions. These come from both immunologic and psychological perspectives. There are known immune differences between populations based upon gender; race; age; body mass index; and even comorbidities, such as whether or not pharmaceutical agents are being taken. From a psychological perspective, an individual's *perception* of stress, rather than the specific stressor alone, has gained increasing importance in naturalistic research studies.[39] Duplicating such perceptions in the laboratory, especially in human studies, will be daunting.

If PNI is to advance as a meaningful discipline in clinical medicine, the previously mentioned challenges must be overcome. It is no longer tenable to use statistical methodology based solely on population analysis that may have a meaningful p-value, but offers little if any direct application to patients. The solution will clearly involve defining criteria, such as biomarkers, that can identify stress-susceptible *individuals* in the long term and higher-risk *subpopulations* in the short term. Such techniques must be able to identify whether stress susceptibility is permanent (genetic), temporary (environmental), or both (eg, moderate genetic susceptibility under severe environmental conditions), as well as make clear the duration and clinical impact of these changes. Just as individual risk for the adverse effects are known to vary, so too can we expect individual responses to specific stress management therapies to vary in effectiveness unless/until we become more effective in our classification of individual stress risk.

REFERENCES

1. Ader R. Psychoneuroimmunology. Ilar J 1998;39(1):27–9.
2. Cohen S. Keynote presentation at the eighth International Congress of behavioral medicine: the Pittsburgh common cold studies: psychosocial predictors of susceptibility to respiratory infectious illness. Int J Behav Med 2005;12(3): 123–31.
3. Agarwal SK, Marshall GD Jr. Stress effects on immunity and its application to clinical immunology. Clin Exp Allergy 2001;31:25–31.
4. Rabin B. Stress: a system of the whole. In: Ader R, editor. Psychoneuroimmunology. 4th edition. New York: Elsevier; 2007. p. 709–22.

5. Webster JI, Tonelli L, Sternberg EM. Neuroendocrine regulation of immunity. Annu Rev Immunol 2002;20:125–63.
6. Koh KB. Emotions and immunity. J Psychosom Res 1998;45:107–15.
7. Scott KM, Von Korff M, Ormel J, et al. Mental disorders among adults with asthma: results from the world mental health survey. Gen Hosp Psychiatry 2007;29:123–33.
8. Roy-Byrne PP, Davidson KW, Kessler RC, et al. Anxiety disorders and comorbid medical illness. Gen Hosp Psychiatry 2008;30:208–25.
9. Lorton D, Lubahn C, Bellinger DL. Potential use of drugs that target neural-immune pathways in the treatment of rheumatoid arthritis and other autoimmune diseases. Curr Drug Targets Inflamm Allergy 2003;2:1–30.
10. Taylor H, Liu J, Wilson G, et al. Distinct component profiles and high risk among African Americans with metabolic syndrome: the Jackson Heart Study. Diabetes Care 2008;31(6):1248–53.
11. Minor DS, Wofford MR, Jones DW. Racial and ethnic differences in hypertension. Curr Atheroscler Rep 2008;10(2):121–7.
12. Maric C. Sex, diabetes and the kidney. Am J Physiol Renal Physiol 2009;296(4): F680–8.
13. Abbas AK, Lichtman AH, Pillai S. Cellular and molecular immunology. 6th edition. Philadelphia: Saunders Elsevier; 2010.
14. Coffman RL. Origins of the T(H)1-T(H)2 model: a personal perspective. Nat Immunol 2006;7:539–41.
15. Sakaguchi S, Miyara M, Costantino CM, et al. FOXP3+ regulatory T cells in the human immune system. Nat Rev Immunol 2010;10(7):490–500.
16. Godbout JP, Glaser R. Stress-induced immune dysregulation: implications for wound healing, infectious disease and cancer. J Neuroimmune Pharm 2006;1:421–7.
17. Marshall GD, Roy SR. Stress and allergic disease. In: Ader R, editor. Psychoneuroimmunology. 4th edition. New York: Elsevier; 2007. p. 799–824.
18. Pant S, Ramaswamy B. Association of major stressors with elevated risk of breast cancer incidence or relapse. Drugs Today (Barc) 2009;45:115–26.
19. Leserman J. Role of depression, stress, and trauma in HIV disease progression. Psychosom Med 2008;70:539–45.
20. Cámara RJ, Ziegler R, Begré S, et al. Swiss Inflammatory Bowel Disease Cohort Study (SIBDCS) group The role of psychological stress in inflammatory bowel disease: quality assessment of methods of 18 prospective studies and suggestions for future research. Digestion 2009;80(2):129–39.
21. Bauer ME, Jeckel CM, Luz C. The role of stress factors during aging of the immune system. Ann N Y Acad Sci 2009;1153:139–52.
22. Gasperin D, Netuveli G, Dias-da-Costa JS, et al. Effect of psychological stress on blood pressure increase: a meta-analysis of cohort studies. Cad Saude Publica 2009;25:715–26.
23. Goddard AW, Ball SG, Martinez J, et al. Current perspectives of the roles of the central norepinephrine system in anxiety and depression. Depress Anxiety 2010; 27(4):339–50.
24. Franklin BA. Impact of psychosocial risk factors on the heart: changing paradigms and perceptions. Phys Sportsmed 2009;37(3):35–7. Review.
25. Glaser R. Stress-associated immune dysregulation and its importance for human health: a personal history of psychoneuroimmunology. Brain Behav Immun 2005; 19:3–11.
26. Yang EV, Glaser R. Stress-associated immunomodulation and its implications for responses to vaccination. Expert Rev Vaccines 2002;1:453–9.

27. Marshall GD. Neuroendocrine mechanisms of immune dysregulation: applications to allergy and asthma. Ann Allergy Asthma Immunol 2004;93(2 Suppl 1): S11–7.
28. Mitsonis CI, Potagas C, Zervas I, et al. The effects of stressful life events on the course of multiple sclerosis: a review. Int J Neurosci 2009;119:315–35.
29. Stojanovich L. Stress and autoimmunity. Autoimmun Rev 2010;9:A271–6.
30. Pouwer F, Kupper N, Adriaanse MC. Does emotional stress cause type 2 diabetes mellitus? A review from the European Depression in Diabetes (EDID) Research Consortium. Discov Med 2010;9:112–8.
31. Freier E, Weber CS, Nowottne U, et al. Decrease of CD4(+)FOXP3(+) T regulatory cells in the peripheral blood of human subjects undergoing a mental stressor. Psychoneuroendocrinology 2010;35:663–73.
32. Calcagni E, Elenkov I. Stress system activity, innate and T helper cytokines, and susceptibility to immune-related diseases. Ann N Y Acad Sci 2006;1069:62–76.
33. Marshall GD. Identifying the stress susceptible patient at risk for inflammatory diseases: an interdisciplinary approach. Expert Rev Clin Immunol 2009;5:119–21.
34. Granger DA, Kivlhigan KT, EL-Sheikh M, et al. Salivary amylase in biobehavioral research: recent developments and applications. Ann N Y Acad Sci 2007;1098: 122–44.
35. Sternthal MJ, Enlow MB, Cohen S, et al. Maternal interpersonal trauma and cord blood IgE levels in an inner-city cohort: a life-course perspective. J Allergy Clin Immunol 2009;124:954–60.
36. Marshall GD, Agarwal SA, Lloyd C, et al. Cytokine dysregulation associated with exam stress in healthy medical students. Brain Behav Immun 1998;12:297–307.
37. Zhang Y, Zhang Y, Miao J, et al. Chronic restraint stress promotes immune suppression through toll-like receptor 4-mediated phosphoinositide 3-kinase signaling. J Neuroimmunol 2008;204:13–9.
38. Xiang L, Marshall GD Jr. Immunomodulatory effects of in vitro stress hormones on FoxP3, Th1/Th2 cytokine and costimulatory molecule mRNA expression in human peripheral blood mononuclear cells. Neuroimmunomodulation 2010;18:1–10.
39. Costa-Pinto FA, Palermo-Neto J. Neuroimmune interactions in stress. Neuroimmunomodulation 2010;17:196–9.

Index

Note: Page numbers of article titles are in **boldface** type.

Immunol Allergy Clin N Am 31 (2011) 141–148
doi:10.1016/S0889-8561(10)00108-6
0889-8561/11/$ – see front matter © 2011 Elsevier Inc. All rights reserved.

immunology.theclinics.com

Moving?

Make sure your subscription moves with you!

To notify us of your new address, find your **Clinics Account Number** (located on your mailing label above your name), and contact customer service at:

Email: journalscustomerservice-usa@elsevier.com

800-654-2452 (subscribers in the U.S. & Canada)
314-447-8871 (subscribers outside of the U.S. & Canada)

Fax number: 314-447-8029

Elsevier Health Sciences Division
Subscription Customer Service
3251 Riverport Lane
Maryland Heights, MO 63043

*To ensure uninterrupted delivery of your subscription, please notify us at least 4 weeks in advance of move.

Printed and bound by CPI Group (UK) Ltd, Croydon, CR0 4YY

03/10/2024

01040447-0014